SO-AAE-123

I

Praise for "Depression in the Young" from:

PARENTS

"Your books should be required reading for every high school and college student and teacher. Thank you for explaining these conditions so clearly!" *Mary Kluesner, Chairperson, SA\VE*

"We are in desperate need of information on childhood depression. This book truly fills the gap; a gift to all families." *Marilyn Koenig, Friends for Survival*

"Your book serves as a guide for the signs of the neurobiological condition that causes many cases of childhood depression." *Tracy Pierson, young woman whose brother suffered from depression*

HEALTH CARE PROFESSIONALS:

"As more people become familiar with treating young bipolar patients with small amounts of lithium, the death rate will be reduced enourmously." *Elisabeth Kubler-Ross, M.D.*

"This book is important for every parent and teacher to read." *Barry D. Garfinkel, M.D., F.R.C.P. (C) Child and Adolescent Psychiatry, Medical School, University of Minnesota.*

TEACHERS:

"This is a very helpful book for parents and teachers who are struggling with these problems in their families and classrooms." *Jo Stewart M.S., English Teacher*

"This is the first book I could truly identify with, as a mother and an educator. Your personal account puts the complexities of brain diseases into an easy to understand format; written from the heart and the mind." *Vicki M. Bresson, SA\VE Board Member*

"Trudy writes with precision and clarity. Her willingness to dig deep into her soul will help others who are looking for guidance." *Robin Blatnik, M.A.E.S., English,Instructor*

Publisher's Note

The information in this book regarding illness is intended to raise the awareness of the symptoms of depression, attention deficit hyperactive disorder, and anxiety disorder in young people, as well as the potentially effective treatments for these conditions. It is not a substitute for the advice and directions of your personal physician. It is not meant to encourage anyone to take any medications or make changes in the way current medications are taken without first consulting your doctor.

Depression in the Young

What We Can Do to Help Them

By Trudy Carlson

FIRST EDITION

Benline Press, Duluth, Minnesota

IV

Copyright 1998 by Trudy Carlson M.S.

ISBN 096424435-7 Library of Congress No. 96-083676

All rights reserved. No part of this book may be reproduced or utilized in any form or by any means, electronic or mechanical, including photocopying, recording or by any information storage and retrieval system, without permission in writing from the publisher. For information address:

Benline Press, 118 N. 60th Avenue East
Duluth, Minnesota 55804

Publisher's Cataloging in Publication Data
Carlson, Trudy M.
Depression in the Young: What We Can Do To Help Them
Includes bibliographical references and Index
1. Depression in children.
2. Depression in children--Treatment
RJ506.D4 618.92/8527 96-083676
096424435-7

Excerpts from "The Good News about Depression" by Mark S. Gold, Copyright ©1984 by Mark S. Gold, Larry Chilnik & Ben Stern. Reprinted by permission of Villard Books, a division of Random House, Inc.

Beck Depression Inventory. Copyright © 1978 by Aaron T. Beck. Reproduced by permission of Publisher, The Psychological Corporation. All rights reserved. "Beck Depression Inventory" and "BDI" are registered trademarks of The Psychological Corporation.

Excerpts from "The Power of Myth" Joseph Campbell & Bill Moyers, © 1988 by Apostrophe S Productions Inc., and Bill Moyers, and Alfred van der Marck Editions Inc., for itself and the estate of Joseph Campbell. Used by permission of Doubleday, a division of Bantam Doubleday Dell Publishing Group Inc.

TABLE OF CONTENTS

ACKNOWLEDGMENT

No book is the product of just one person. My heartfelt gratitude goes to everyone who contributed to it. I want to thank those individuals who read this work in manuscript form at various stages. They include: Roseann Biever, Caroline Carlson, Lu Harter, Char Gallian, Margaret Kinetz, Monica Natzel, Carol Nord, Rod Nord, Jo Stewart, Nancy Scheftner, Dr. Elisabeth Kubler-Ross, Dr. Barry Garfinkel, Dr. Kenneth Irons, Dr. Jerome Kwako, Carol Michaelson, Eileen Gannon, and Dr. Carrie Borchardt.

I would like to make special mention of Kristen Oberg, Patt Jackson and Robin Blatnik, the editors of the book, whose skill and encouragement helped to make it what it is. Their sustained commitment to this project is the kind of help writers dream of receiving, but never expect to get.

I wish to express appreciation to all the works that are quoted in this book. The list of these are contained in the bibliography.

There can be no full accounting of the debt I owe to the scores of people who contributed to this project by giving me advice and/or technical assistance. They include: Dr. Aaron Beck, Dr. Kenneth Broman, Joseph Gallian, Sheldon T. Aubut, Ann Sanford, Melanie Horn, Mary Kluesner, Marilyn Koenig, Tracy Pierson, Vicki Blesson. Special thanks to my brothers and sisters who helped me in a number of ways.

The cover is designed by David Garon, and the painting on the cover is by Garry Carlson.

Preface

On May 31, 1989, Benjamin Drew Carlson, aged fourteen, killed himself. In 1995 <u>The Suicide of My Son: A Story of Childhood Depression</u> was published. The book is both the story of Ben's life and the story behind the story. Part I shows how his depression, ADHD, and anxiety disorder manifest at various stages of his life, from infancy to adolescents. Part II gives the scientific information on the symptoms, treatment of depression and anxiety, and fact about suicide in the young.

Response to this book has been favorable. When this book has been displayed at conferences for parents, teachers, counselors and therapists, a frequent comment is that people like to have books that are light weight, easy to pick up, carry in a purse or brief case. Consequently, while continuing to publish the original volume, the decision was made to also present it as two separate, smaller books. Part I is now published as <u>Ben's Story: The Symptoms of Depression, ADHD and Anxiety that Caused His Suicide</u>. Part II is now published as <u>Depression in the Young: What We Can do to Help Them.</u>

If You're So Smart, How Come Your Son Is Dead?

That is the question I felt everyone was thinking but was too polite to ask. I taught college classes in child and adolescent psychology, developmental psychology, as well as personality and mental health. How could it be that a well-informed, concerned parent raised a child who would later commit suicide?

When I began to write the story of my son's life and death, I decided to include a chapter with this title. I wanted to explain how it is that knowing about depression and doing everything you can to help a person cope does not guarantee that everyone with a complex, serious form of depression will survive.

Ben's Story: The Symptoms of Childhood Depression, ADHD, and Anxiety Causing His Suicide describes how these conditions manifested themselves in various stages of his life. As I began to search for answers about Ben's life and death, and for ways to prevent this tragedy in other families, an idea for a chapter turned into a separate manuscript. The story of the complex and biological nature of depression and anxiety in young people simply can not be effectively told in one brief chapter.

Depression is a painful illness. Certain cancer patients who had also experienced depression were asked which pain was more bearable. Overwhelmingly they answered that they would rather cope with the physical pain of cancer than the pain of depression. Anxiety, too, is painful as well as frightening. Anyone who has ever experienced a panic attack can attest to anxiety's interference with the simple task of daily living.

My primary goal in writing is to help reduce the unnecessary suffering of depression and anxiety. We know that pain and suffering are a natural part of our lives; without them there would also be no joy. Those who experience the pain of anxiety can learn to use the unavoidable portion of this condition as a means to develop more depth to their personality. On the other hand, the experience of avoidable pain is generally pointless and does not enrich one's life. Avoidable pain occurs when we fail to see how depression and anxiety operate in our lives, and when we fail to seek effective ways of dealing with them.

We live in a time when effective treatment for depression and anxiety are available. The good news is becoming more well known as adults who experience the pain of these conditions are willing to share what their lives have taught them. The good news is also being spread by doctors and other scientists who share what they have learned about effective treatments.

My son's life, and the lessons I have learned since his death, have taught me a great deal. My special purpose is to focus on children and young adults, and to show parents, teachers, and counselors how they can help these students in easy, low-cost ways. We have done much in the way of treating adult depression and anxiety, but many of our young people remain misunderstood, misdiagnosed and untreated. Reading these pages can give hope to worried parents, guidance to concerned teachers, counselors, and a lifetime of benefit to the younger people who silently suffer.

Cognitive therapy is one of several new methods especially designed to treat the symptoms of depression. Having the individual engage in experiments that disprove their negative assumptions about themselves, combined with the use of homework tasks, makes cognitive therapy ideally suited for groups of school-aged persons. Cognitive-behavioral therapy has great potential to counteract the greatest risk factor for suicide -- hopelessness.

Anxiety is now recognized as a dangerous factor for persons with serious depression. New research indicates that the presence of panic attacks is highly predictive of those depressed persons in imminent danger of suicide attempts. The same type of medicine used to treat depression also helps to decrease biologically based anxiety. Although some of the cognitive-behavior techniques can also help decrease anxiety, there are other special techniques that can be taught to these groups. New coping skills would benefit those interested in improving the quality of life in these highly stressful times in which we all live.

Medication plays a key role in the treatment of serious forms of depression and anxiety. As the owner/operator of health care facilities for handicapped adults, I am familiar with a wide range of medicines including those for the treatment of depression. But it is my personal experience as a mother that has most significantly motivated me to seek the latest research regarding the most effective ways to utilize these medicines. My chapter on medications is easy to understand, and incorporates my experience as well as clinical findings of current research. An appendix also lists further sources of help and information.

Finally, the chapter on suicide deals with the complex nature of this tragedy. It shows how prevention lies in treating the illness that causes the death. Proper diagnosis of any illness involves objective analysis of data relative to the symptom. Screening young people with easy to complete self-report forms which can also be self-scored, is a fast, inexpensive way to identify young people at risk. Because this type of screening could take just minutes and cost next to nothing, it can easily be incorporated several times a year from middle elementary to college students. Self screening for depression is not much different from taking your own temperature, and is no more mysterious.

When I was a child, the big medical challenge was the prevention and treatment of polio. The Mother's March of Dimes was a grass-roots effort to raise the money needed to do the necessary scientific research which enabled us to develop a vaccine against this disease. Today, one of our biggest medical challenges is the prevention and treatment of depression. However, we do not need to raise money to do scientific research; major drug companies have already spent the money needed to produce medicines with proven efficacy.

Caring adults genuinely want to help young people whose depressed mood interferes with their ability to concentrate on their school work and which makes them moody and irritable. Parents, teachers, health care professionals and all concerned adults need to arm themselves with awareness of symptoms as they appear in children, because depression looks different in young people than it does in adults. And they need to become knowledgeable of the treatments that are currently available with proven effectiveness. The real tragedy of depression in the young exists only when effective treatments are not used, and children are allowed to experience easily avoidable suffering.

Depression in Perspective

B efore focusing on how we can help our young people with depression, it is important to start with a fundamental understanding of the nature of this condition. In the past when a young person showed signs of depression, there was an over-emphasis on looking at what parents were doing wrong or failed to do right. Not only did that often prove to be unproductive in helping the child, but it obviously would not prevent most parents from viewing the young person's depression objectively.

This chapter focuses on the biological nature of depression. Important environmental factors are put in the more relevant context of overall, historical terms rather than the personal characteristics of individual families. Depression is no one's fault. Excessive guilt will not arise from a logical examination of truly significant factors that produce depression.

My grief following Ben's death led me to spend a lot of time reading about depression and suicide. I discovered it is nearly impossible to predict when someone is going to attempt suicide. Effective prevention needs to focus on treatment of the conditions most frequently associated with suicide, namely depression and anxiety. Both conditions are important to understand, but since depression is a factor in at least 80 percent of suicides, I will start with it.

INCIDENCE OF DEPRESSION

The major obstacle to overcome in any discussion of depression is the idea that it is a rare illness. Depression is anything but rare. Although it is fairly uncommon for the condition to be fatal (only about 15% of severally depressed persons end their lives), the illness in its milder forms is both common and painful. Psychiatrist and author Dr. David Burns (1980) writes, "Depression has been called the world's number one public health problem." Various books and articles give different statistics on exactly how many people are affected by mood disorders.

This is what we are dealing with today. "A 1986 study of Minnesota high school students reveals that 39% suffer from mild to severe depression." ("Adolescent," 1986). Dr. Mark Gold (1987), biopsychiatrist and author of The Good News About Depression, writes that the findings for college students is similar to what is found in high school. Gold states, "One out of three college students will have experienced a unipolar or bipolar episode by the time he or she has graduated."

What is the rate for adults? Dr. Gerald Klerman (1984), eminent psychiatrist and author of books on interpersonal psychotherapy for depression, wrote that "Although only a small minority of individuals experiences depressive symptoms that meet the criteria of a clinical disorder, many more experience depressive moods; about 40 percent of the population report feeling depression, disappointment and unhappiness in a year."

As we begin to realize that four out of every ten people high school age and over have some level of depression, it becomes clear why depression is the number one public health problem in the world. When you develop an awareness of the symptoms of this illness, you get an understanding of what is wrong with so many of us today. You generally hear experts talk about the incidence of depression as 10 percent. That figure refers to people with severe (clinical) depression. Ten percent of our adolescent and adult population is clinically depressed, while 30 percent has milder forms of depression; which gives a total of 40 percent.

If the incidence of mild to severe depression in teens and adults is 40%, what is the rate of depression in children? It is a hard question to answer. Dr. Gold (1987, p. 282) tells us, "Twenty years ago, psychiatrists believed that depression in childhood did not and could not exist. Now experts in child health are sounding an alarm." Parents would like to believe depression is not as high for children as it is for adolescents and adults, but experts tell us children are actually the population which has seen the greatest increase in recent years.

Getting an accurate figure on the occurrence of childhood depression is currently impossible. Most depression for all age groups goes undiagnosed. We do not screen youngsters for this very common condition. Psychiatrists can only guess at the incidence of childhood depression. In their landmark book on childhood depression, Why Johnny Isn't Crying, McKnew, Cytryn and Yahrens (1983) estimate the rate of severe depression in children ranges from 5 percent to 10 percent. This estimate for children is not that different from the data on adults -- about 10 percent suffer from severe depression.

McKnew (1983) and his colleagues believe the incidence of severe depression in children to be "from three to more than six million American children," most of which "goes unrecognized and untreated." As distressing as these figures are, they do not reflect the incidence of milder forms of depression. The amount of mild depression in children may be an additional 30 percent, the same as it is for adolescents and adults. Dr. Gold (1987) makes this comment about the lack of diagnosis in children: "The terrible truth (is childhood depression) has caught psychiatrists and pediatricians by surprise."

How is it the general public and often the medical profession have not only failed to recognize the condition but also underestimate how many young people are affected by it today? One of the reasons may be that the amount of depression seems to fluctuate at different times in history and the current high rates of mood disorders have just taken everyone by surprise.

HISTORICAL PERSPECTIVE

We do not have to go very far back to see another time in our history when depression was common. The pattern after World War I is similar in some respects to the pattern experienced since World War II. The first World War was the famous war to end all wars. The Roaring Twenties which followed the victory for the Allies was a particularly optimistic time. This optimism not only gave hope for a peaceful future under a League of Nations but a time of unlimited economic opportunities. The 1929 stock market crash ushered in an end to the exaggerated optimism. Not only was there an economic depression, but the people felt depressed. Physicians and psychiatrists began to report a widespread incidence of symptoms of what they continued to call melancholia (depression). The losses people had incurred in their lives (loss of financial security, loss of work activity, perhaps loss of their home, etc.) and the dramatic changes they were then forced to make were the cause of changed mood.

Not all loss and change results in depression. It is only when loss and change feels purposeless, meaningless, and when there is little optimism for the future that depression occurs. World War II also created its share of both change and loss, but the war solved our economic depression and lifted the nation out of its psychological depression. During the war our country busily pursued purposeful, meaningful activity, something it had not been able to do during the Depression of the 1930's.

The years after the Great War were called the Fabulous Fifties, a time of economic prosperity and stability. Because U.S. factories were not bombed during the war, America was in a position to make the products needed throughout many parts of the world. It was also a time of low rates of depression and low rates of suicide.

The decade following the bombing of Hiroshima brought a gradual proliferation of weapons and the slow realization that we were living in dangerous times. Born in 1944, I grew up in the 50's and 60's and came to know it was possible for a bomb like that to fall on us as well, destroying life as we know it. Poets and artists often become alert to change before the general public. W. H. Auden's poem, The Age of Anxiety, published in 1947, captured the feeling of the later 50's. The threat of possible annihilation which the atomic age produced was constant and something we could do little about.

My daughter is a child of the 70's and 80's. When I described to her what it was like to grow up with the anxiety of the nuclear bomb, she described to me in elegant terms why we have now shifted from a post war Age of Anxiety into an Age of Depression. She says it is almost irrelevant whether or not we have a war between a few superpowers possessing nuclear weapons. Indeed, the general lessening of tension between the former communist countries and the democracies of the West has not decreased the sense of danger felt by her generation. There is no exaggerated optimism in the 90's following the end of the cold war similar to what was experienced following the other major wars of this century. She cites overpopulation, nuclear accidents, nuclear waste and a number of other problems relating to the ecology of the planet which, from her perspective, make our destruction seem inevitable.

The words she spoke to me in our kitchen are echoed in the work of psychiatrist and author, Anthony Stevens (1989). He writes:

> If we continue as we are, the possibility of nuclear catastrophe is matched only by the certainty of ecological disaster. The explosive increase in world population, infinite problems of providing enough food, the rapid growth of industrial pollution, the poisoning of the atmosphere, the oceans, lakes, and streams, the destruction of the tropical rain forests and the countryside, the elimination of animal species, the occurrence of disasters in nuclear power stations, the disposal of radioactive waste, the spread of nuclear weapons, the exhaustion of the earth's resources, the turning of productive land into desert -- all threaten to make life on this planet insupportable in a century's time.

There is a joke going around which says, "The only people who aren't depressed are the people who do not know what is going on."

Our nation has not experienced a major economic depression lately. Instead, it has protracted economic stress caused by a combination of the high cost of living with reduction in high paying jobs. Families make substantial investment in their children's education, only to discover that returns on that investment in terms of a good job are illusive. Can this generation as easily obtain the standard of living their parents had? Perhaps not.

Another factor creating the second epidemic of depression in this century relates to social upheaval. Canadian research indicates that social upheaval "results in the breakdown of social cohesion and increases social disorganization, which is reflected in increased rates of mental illness" (Klerman, 1984). Loss is a factor in social change. During times of dramatic change, social structure and traditional patterns are altered. Depression is more likely during transitions when familiar patterns are gone and a new way of life has not yet been established.

The dramatic changes since World War II have been the subject of many magazine articles and television documentaries. We feel it in every aspect of our lives: in the communications sector with the advent of satellites, in health with the development of new life-saving procedures, in politics as empires break down creating opportunities as well as instabilities. With just these few examples illustrating change, we can appreciate why stress is an important factor in recent decades.

Dr. Gold (1987), like so many others, describes our era as marked by extreme and exceedingly rapid changes.

Throughout the world, we are in an era of social, political and technological revolution. The science we learn in school is invalid by the time we reach adulthood. The computer is second nature to our children, but to many parents and grandparents this fundamental new tool will remain a mystery. Children have power and independence unheard of just a short time ago. Teenagers murder. Teenagers commit suicide. Life expectancy is longer, but money runs out. Conquer heart disease and what do you get? Cancer. Horrible diseases like AIDS appear out of nowhere.

When I was a child, my parents were worried about polio. Now, we worry about Lyme's Disease. We may have eradicated smallpox with our vaccines, but there is no vaccine for AIDS. Over optimism that disease can be eradicated through scientific discovery has been tempered by the reality that occurs with the arrival of new diseases. And as antibiotics become less effective against more resilient strains of bacteria, old diseases once again become a problem. We are no more able to eliminate disease than we are of eliminating war. The changing realities of life may be one reason for the rise of depressive illness in the 1970's and 80's. Gold (1987, p. 190) writes, "Depression is believed to be on the rise worldwide, perhaps even epidemic."

Our shift from an Age of Anxiety (the term used to describe the era follow the dropping of the atomic bomb) to an Age of Depression (the term that could describe the era of slowly declining economic prosperity for the average wage earner, slowly rising cost of living, and accelerating demands to cope with continuous change) produces a general sense of loss. We may be living in a time when some of the changes are not viewed as purposeful or meaningful and there is little optimism for the future. We have been taught to think that change means progress, and progress is good; however, progress is a two-edged sword that cuts both ways. Adapting to fast-paced, dramatic changes has made us feel vulnerable.

No one can be absolutely certain why depression is so common in the last part of the Twentieth Century. Many theories have been suggested.

A greater gap between expectations and fulfillment than in previous generations, increased drug use and greater mobility, all have been proposed as possible reasons for the increase in the 1970's and 80's. Some even suggest that a change in biological factors is at work, but conclusive evidence for any of these theories is not yet at hand (Goode, 1990, p. 53).

While scientists try to discover the cause of history's latest rise in the incidence of depression, I would emphasize one thing to anyone coping with this problem: If you have this illness or someone you love has this condition, it is not your fault. Whether the depression is due to some general, overriding environmental factor, such as the stress of life in the last part of this century, or if the depression is more related to genetic factors, as it was for my son, or if the depression is caused by a combination of environmental factors and genetic predisposition, which is often the case, it still is not your fault. Depression is similar to many other illnesses such as cancer, heart disease, or diabetes. Like them, there seems to be genetic factors or environmental/lifestyle factors or (most commonly) a combination of both the genetic and environmental/lifestyle factors which affect the formation of the illness. For example, cigarette smoking is a lifestyle factor that can affect cancer and heart disease. Obesity resulting from overeating can also contribute to the development of those same illnesses, as well as diabetes. Yet, genetics is a strong factor in predicting who is likely to be at risk for developing cancer, heart disease, and diabetes. Genetics and lifestyle all combine to produce risk.

No one would blame the victim of cancer, heart disease, or diabetes for their conditions, nor would anyone blame their parents. The same should be said about depression. If you are depressed or your child experiences depressive illness, it is not anyone's fault that this condition exists. Once this fact is fully understood and appreciated, there will be less guilt associated with depressive illness and more willingness to seek treatment. Depression is now being recognized as a physiological problem: e.g., a problem caused by neurotransmitters and/or hormones. As we come to know the biology of this illness, it will allow us to be more objective about the condition, seeing it as a medical condition, not a sign of personal weakness.

Today's challenge for the person who has the condition, or their loved ones, is to recognize depression as a treatable medical condition. The optimistic news about depression is that the National Institute of Mental Health has done a nationwide study which has determined the existence of a number of highly effective treatments. The problem with depression lies not so much in its treatment (the success rate is at least 80 percent) but in lack of recognition or diagnosis of the condition as a treatable illness. Sometimes persons with the condition fail to seek medical help; other times they go to their doctor, telling them of their symptoms, and the physician does not diagnosis it. This means we, as the general public, need to know the symptoms of depression if we are to cope with the number one public health problem.

TYPES OF DEPRESSIVE ILLNESS

To get a fuller perspective on depression, it is helpful to include a description of the many forms it can take. I will use Ben as an example when it applies because, unfortunately for him, he exemplifies several different forms of depressive illness. I know I have his blessing in doing this, because once when I was teaching an adult evening class, I asked Ben if I could use one of his experiences as an example. His response was: "If it can be used to help someone else, go right ahead."

Dysthymia

Dysthymia is a chronic depressive condition in which people feel out of sorts all of the time. They are not deeply depressed, but neither do they feel good. Weather makes a useful analogy to describe the mood of people suffering from dysthymia. Their mood is not like a thunderstorm (dark and dangerous), but neither do they experience blue skies and sunshine. One could say their world is gray and overcast most of the time. They are generally unhappy, although they may put on a smile to allow others to feel more comfortable. Virginia Commonwealth University clinical psychologist James McCullough says, "Researchers estimate that nearly 9 million Americans are locked in dysthymia's dispiriting grip, `It's like a low-grade infection....Dysthymics never really feel good' (Goode, 1990, p. 51).

Ben had dysthymia. Depression was a fairly constant condition throughout his childhood. Ben told his psychiatrist he felt depressed all of his life. His medical records include this notation: "He states that he does not remember a time when he has felt happy most of the time."

Dysthymia is not just a minor depressive problem. A booklet published by the National Institute of Mental Health states,

Some people with dysthymia also have episodes of major depression, their symptoms becoming dramatically more severe for a while and then returning to their usual reduced level. These people are said to have double depression, that is, dysthymia plus major depression. Individuals with double depression are at much higher risk for recurring episodes of major depression, so careful treatment and follow-up are very important (Sargent, 1989a).

SAD (Seasonal Affective Disorder)

Living in northern Minnesota, I have been especially interested in one of the newer discoveries about depression. What we always called "the winter blahs," are scientifically defined as Seasonal Affective Disorder. Researchers indicate that for people suffering from SAD "despair sets in with the disappearance of the lingering daylight hours of summer and persists for as long as short days and the cold winter sun remain. As spring returns, however, patients with SAD feel their energy return. Their desolation lifts and their lives return to normal." (Goode, 1990, p. 51).

There may be a correlation between this pattern in humans and what animals experience in winter. People with SAD, like hibernating animals, "crave sleep, they also binge on carbohydrates, gaining weight from October through March." (Gelman, 1987, p. 54). The over-eating and over-sleeping with SAD is interesting because people with other common forms of depressive conditions under-eat and lack the ability to sleep.

What causes SAD? "The culprit may be a sleep inducing hormone called melatonin, which is produced in the dark. Or, as other researchers now believe, SAD may be a biological phenomenon left over from prehistoric man, who conserved energy during the cold winter months when food was scarce." (Gelman, 1987, p. 54).

People with seasonal depression are helped by sitting close to a bank of lights that emit rays similar to natural light. Patients in the past sat 3 feet away from the light and stayed there for 2 hours. If you put the same light 15 inches away, you may only need a 30 minute treatment. Some people find the new desk-top lights convenient. One-half of people with winter depression are bipolar (manic-depression), whereas people with unipolar depression may experience changes in mood in the spring and fall when in the rate change of sun light is at it greatest.

Ben's psychiatrist told me he probably had seasonal depression. She noted his increase in symptoms during the colder months and a rise in energy as warmer weather came.

Some people with SAD move closer to the equator for part of the winter. I think of our vacations in Florida each winter and feel they may have done him more good than I realized at the time.

Reactive Depression

Reactive depressions are a reaction to an event or condition in one's life. These depressions can be severe, but most people recover without necessarily experiencing other recurrences. Often it is a loss of some kind. Grief has been interpreted as a normal form of reactive depression.

Recurring Unipolar Depression

People with recurring unipolar depressions (periods of low mood wthout obvious manic episodes) feel low with or without stressors in the environment. These people have normal moods much of the time, but have a number of depressive episodes during their lifetime. The National Institute of Mental Health describes the symptoms:

1. *persistent sadness*
2. *low energy*
3. *loss of interest in activities*
4. *feeling of hopelessness, guilt, worthlessness*
5. *difficulty with sleep, memory, concentration*
6. *chronic aches or persistent bodily symptoms*
      (Sargent, 1989a).

Unipolar depression is especially important to understand simply because it is the most common form of depression.

Bipolar Illness

Victims of bipolar illness (also known as manic-depressive disorder) enjoy normal moods some of the time. When they have bouts of this illness, they alternate between depression and mania. When depressed, they experience symptoms of unipolar depression, but persons with bipolar illness also have times when they are high or manic. The National Institute of Mental Health (NIMH) says that when persons with bipolar are in a manic phase of the cycle, they typically have:

1. *increased energy*
2. *decreased need for sleep*
3. *increased risk-taking*
4. *feelings of mood elevation or irritability*
5. *aggressive response to frustration.*
   (Sargent, 1989,a, p. 20).

Bipolar illness comes in two forms.People with bipolar I have manic episodes that can be extreme. During these highs, they have an unrealistic belief in their own abilities; they may incur horrendous debts and make poor business decisions. They show an increase in talking, as well as physical and social activity. People around them see them as "hyper." There can be an increase in sexual activity to the point of promiscuity. People tend to overlook the painful or harmful consequences of their manic behavior. Their high energy and possibly aggressive response to frustration may even result in breaking the law and landing in jail. All of this may be associated with loss of friends, family, and employment. Not all people with bipolar I have all of these symptoms and most are helped with lithium. If you took chemistry in school you saw lithium on the chart of basic natural elements. Lithium has proven to be very effective in stabilizing the highs for persons with bipolar illness. Besides lithium, physicians are now using some of the medications traditionally used to control epilepsy for people with bipolar illness. Some bipolar patients are helped by carbamazapine, others are helped by valproate.

All indications were that Ben did not have Bipolar I. Ben's illness corresponds to the symptoms of Bipolar II. His highs did not get extremely high; his manic episodes would have been called hypomanic (small manic). For example, his increased talking was mildly disruptive to family conversations, but a casual observer might not have seen him as excessively talkative. His increased physical activity caused him to get too carried away during roughhouse play. Ben loved to wrestle with his dad and when he was younger his father would just hold him down when Ben got a little out of control. But during the last year, there were several times in which Ben, quite unintentionally, hurt his dad when he got carried away when they wrestled.

Our daughter, Caroline, discovered early in her childhood that playing with Ben was often difficult if not impossible, because he would get physically out of control. His hypomanic behavior meant that he was not hyper all of the time, but there were times when his behavior was excessive. He did not seem to be able to control this. He never intended to hurt anyone and was always remorseful or confused as to what had come over him.

Whenever I would read those neat lists of manic behaviors contrasted to depression, I was always a little frustrated because it seemed to me that Ben was both manic and depressed at the same time. I have since learned that 2/3 of people with bipolar illness experience mixed states. Dr. Kay Jamison writes, "Mixed states represent a critical combination of dysphoric mood (anxiety plus depression), depressed thought combined with an exceptionally perturbed, agitated and unpleasant physical state that is usually accompanied by a heightened energy level and increased impulsivity." (Lifesaver, Summer, 1994). It is interesting to note that there is a high rate of attempted suicide during mixed states.

MULTIPLICITY OF DEPRESSIVE CONDITIONS

In this short look at the various ways depression manifests itself, it is clear the term "depression" is not just one illness but a cluster of conditions. These conditions overlap, and it is possible, if not common, for one person to have a number of them rather than just one. For example, I saw Ben as having bipolar II, and his therapist was able to identify the dysthymia and seasonal depression. Scientists call Ben's combination (dysthymia plus bipolar II) cyclothymia. Dr. Gold (1987) writes that "cyclothymics come from bipolar families." Our son had a number of overlapping conditions, but what is paradoxical is that, to the casual observer, this boy with a ready smile did not seem depressed at all. He, like perhaps as many as 40 percent of children and adolescents with mild to severe depression, was not seen as having a medical condition requiring help.

The Symptoms of Depression in the Young

W hy are we so blind to childhood depression? McKnew, Cytryn and Yahraes (1983) give us their opinion:

> Perhaps the biggest reason is that many depressed children are often the 'nicest' boys and girls on the block and the best behaved kids in school. Go into a classroom and you'll find that the kids in the back rows are the quiet ones, the ones that don't give anyone any trouble, though we know now that many of them are depressed . . . Unless you know a depressed child quite well and are really looking for signs of depression, you probably won't notice anything wrong.

Depression in children does not always look like depression in adults. Depression in youngsters and adults is fundamentally the same illness, but depressed young people rarely have long, sad faces. They frequently have beautiful wide smiles, trying hard not to be a burden to others, attempting to make the best of their painful lives. If we use only the list of adult symptoms, we will miss the vast majority of children and adolescents suffering from depression.

Lists of symptoms of depression in youngsters have been proposed in the past. Often these lists emphasize changes in the child's behavior, but I do not always find lists that emphasize change to be helpful. For example, children with dysthymia are always feeling somewhat blue. Their depression is not a change in behavior, it is the way they feel every day of their lives. Furthermore, children such as Ben who have bipolar illness have a condition with a very early onset. These children have behaviors, body complaints, frequent illnesses, and mood problems throughout their lives. Their depression is not a change; it is the way they have always been.

Children with recurring unipolar depression, on the other hand, *do* have normal mood most of the time. A change in mood does signal the onset of a bout with depression for them. I do not want to discount the value of using a change in behavior as useful in diagnosing depression. I just wish to point out that "change" shouldn't be exclusively used as a criteria in defining depression.

This list by Dr. Carl P. Malmquist of the University of Minnesota avoids referring to change. His symptom list describing childhood depression includes:

1. *Persistent sadness, in contrast to the temporary unhappy moods that normally occur in all children from time to time.*
2. *Low self-concept.*
3. *Provocative, aggressive behavior, or other behavior that leads people to reject or avoid the child.*

4. Proneness to be disappointed easily when things do not go exactly as planned.

5. Physical complaints such as headaches, stomach aches, sleep problems or fatigue, similar to those experienced by depressed adults.

Using Ben as an example where appropriate, I will expand on these five symptoms and then list some which other experts have noted.

1. Persistent sadness, in contrast to the temporary unhappy moods that normally occur in all children from time to time.

What are the conditions that might cause persistent sadness? Children with dysthymia suffer from chronic low mood. Children who suffer from recurring unipolar depression may have the first episode of that condition when they are quite young. Children with bipolar illness have a cyclical condition. Although they will feel normal some of the time, high moods alternate with periods of feeling low. Finally, children who experience a loss of some kind may be beginning a reactive depression that warrants attention. Any child whose sadness persists over a few weeks should be considered for some sort of treatment.

2. Low Self-concept

Depressed children typically have problems with self-esteem. It is a mistake to assume their low self-esteem is always a direct result of environmental factors. Even when parents are very loving and careful to avoid criticizing the child, the depressive illness itself can produce an attitude of self-criticism and low self-esteem for the youngster.

Some depressed children have an overly-sensitive disposition which causes them to interpret any general comment as a criticism. This overly sensitive reaction also interferes with their willingness to ask for help in the classroom. This over-sensitivity results in the perception that other children are picking on them, when in fact this is not true. Ben perceived lots of bullies in the school yard that probably did not exist; playing with neighborhood children often ended with Ben crying and returning home. His over-sensitivity meant he cried easily and generally had problems getting along with peers. Again, the child's overly-sensitive nature may not have anything to do with the actions of parents who may be doing everything they can to help the child feel confident and secure.

3. *Provocative, aggressive behavior, or other behavior that lead people to reject or avoid the child.*

Our daughter learned early in her childhood that Ben was difficult to play with. He would provoke disputes between them. Caroline also noted that when he became aggressive he would either lash out at others or inflict self-injury, such as biting himself. She and her playmates included Ben in their play some of the time, but because they knew that excluding him would mean they could play peacefully, they frequently chose to avoid him.

Ben had marked increases in anger and aggressive behavior when he reached fourth grade. He verbalized his anger, and broke things like pens and pencils. He also did damage in the house by carving on woodwork and defacing furniture. When Ben began seeing a psychiatrist, he mentioned that "his feeling of depression had been worse since about fourth grade." The paradox of the anger expressed by someone with depression is that some of it seems legitimate. Depressed children have every right to feel angry at being misunderstood. They have a right to feel angry at being expected to do things they simply are not able to do. Ben found deep breathing and relaxation methods helpful in controlling his angry feelings.

4. Proneness to be disappointed easily when things do not go exactly as planned.

Ben had a very low tolerance for frustration. When putting together a puzzle, he often pounded on a piece if it did not fit. He did the same to other toys when they did not perform as he wanted. When we would go on a family outing and there was a change or delay in plans, he easily became upset. I have wondered if this proneness to express disappointment is a forerunner to hopelessness and helplessness. Persons with depression often have errors in their thinking which lead them to be more pessimistic than others.

5. *Physical complaints such as headaches, stomach aches, sleep problems, or fatigue, similar to those experienced by depressed adults.*

Physical pain is a common indicator of childhood depression. People do not generally think of bodily pain in conjunction with depression, but it can be an important symptom. Ben told me about the pains in his arms and legs, but at the time I assumed it was the beginning of childhood arthritis, a condition my husband had when he was a child. I never thought of it as a symptom of depression. Headache pain may be especially important. Ben's childhood was plagued by frequent, painful headaches. Researchers have found that persons who experience frequent migraines have a suicide rate three times higher than people who do not.

Depressed children not only have various aches and pains, but are also frequently ill. This may be due to the effect their depression is having on the immune system. As one person said, "When you are depressed, nothing works well." This includes the immune system. The frequent illness some depressed children have contributes to the aches and pains they experience.

One of the hallmarks of depression is sleep abnormalities. Trouble with sleep can either involve insomnia -- difficulty falling asleep or staying asleep; or the opposite -- sleeping too much. Some children are energized at night and then chronically tired during the day, which adds to their problem with concentration and alertness in school. Ben's difficulties with sleep showed up immediately in infancy, and he did not sleep through the night until he was in his second or third year. Problems with sleep continued throughout his life, and he reported feeling tired at school.

6. Inability to concentrate

To Dr. Malmquist's list of symptoms of childhood depression I would add the inability to concentrate. Depressed children have trouble with schoolwork. Psychiatrist and author, Dr. Mark Gold writes about the reciprocal connection between depression and school difficulties in a paragraph headed "Learning Disabilities = Depression, Depression = Learning Disabilities." He says,

> Psychologist David Goldstein conducted a five-year study of 159 learning-disabled children in Philadelphia and found that nearly all of them were depressed. The school problems caused the depression in most of them; but for about one-third, depression produced the school problems.

(Gold, 1987)

Scientists have discovered that the limbic system of the brain is of great importance to a person's learning ability. They also hypothesize that depression is a problem of the limbic system. Little wonder depressed children have learning problems! They may not be able to follow what their teachers say; consequently they do not perform to their potential.

There are a number of factors that facilitate the vicious circle regarding learning problems and depression. First of all, depressed persons of any age have difficulty concentrating. Add to this a phenomena common in animals as well as in persons called "learned helplessness." Learned helplessness occurs when people or animals find themselves in highly stressful or painful situations which they can neither get out of nor manage to cope with successfully. Children with learning problems are in the classic situation which produces learned helplessness. They are forced to be in a school situation they cannot escape from or cope with successfully. It's easy to see why children with learning problems may begin to feel helpless and hopeless. Ben had both manic-depressive illness and an attention deficit disorder. Either one would have created some problems for him in school; together they served to make his experience with school impossible.

7. *Energy fluctuations*

The energy levels of depressed children can fluctuate from normal to hyperactivity and then to sluggishness. Parents find themselves alternating between wanting the child to settle down, and then later wishing the child would do something other than just vegetating in front of the television set. If the child is over-watching TV and not enjoying more active games or hobbies with friends, this may be a clue to some level of depression.

Energy fluctuations are especially true for children with bipolar illness. Pioneer psychiatrist in the treatment of bipolar illness and author Dr. Ronald Fieve (1975) describes bipolar children this way: "Bursts of aggressiveness and frantic activity may alternate with periods of sluggish passivity in a way that resembles the periodic fluctuations of adult moodswings." It is important to suspect bipolar illness in young children because Dr. Gold (1987) states, "many earlier-onset depressions are now believed to be bipolar II depressions."

8. *Eating problems*

Another hallmark of depression is eating abnormalities. The child will either eat too little, consequently becoming thin, or eat too much and carry extra weight. Although Ben ate only small quantities of formula as a newborn, he ate frequently and had normal weight. Throughout most of his life Ben struggled with overeating which is consistent with bipolar II. From his work with young patients, Dr. Charles Popper (1990) writes, "appetite and body weight may exhibit marked fluctuations in bipolar children." Dr. Gold (1987) also cites bipolar II as the type of depression with "reverse" symptoms. Patients tend to oversleep rather than have difficulty sleeping and tend to "eat and eat instead of losing their appetites." The connection between eating problems and depressive illness makes me wonder how many overweight children are suffering from an undiagnosed case of depressive illness.

9. Bladder and Bowel Problems

Bedwetting is mentioned by many psychiatrists including Drs. Gold and Fieve. It is mentioned in relationship to both anxiety and depression. Ben was toilet trained at 2 1/2, but bedwetting started at age five. Nothing we tried was successful in treating this problem. Not every child who has bedwetting episodes is depressed or anxious. But if a parent or doctor sees a cluster of symptoms indicative of either anxiety or depression in addition to the bedwetting, it is possible the wetting is part of either of them. Dr. Klerman also notes that constipation is a common experience in persons with depression. Ben had problems with this from infancy. Not only was it another physical symptom for him to contend with, but treating it was unpleasant.

10. Excessive fearfulness

Fear is one of the major symptoms of anxiety disorder. Because anxiety most often accompanies depression, it is useful to include it as a symptom commonly found in depressed young people. The world is a scary place for depressed children who also suffer from anxiety. It is filled with danger and menace. It puzzles parents to see excessive fearfulness in their child when they are providing the youngster with a safe and secure environment. This certainly was the case with our family. I thought it would be possible to teach Ben to be unafraid by being calm myself and by giving him information that demonstrated the safety of the situation. Although those strategies are generally advisable and I had some success, I was unable to calm those fears completely.

11. Impulsivity

Impulsivity -- acting without thinking about the consequences -- is a major characteristic of children with an attention deficit but is also found in some youngsters with depression. This is especially true of children with bipolar (manic-depressive) illness. Scientific evidence is mounting that bipolar depression is genetically determined. Dr. Gold (1987, p.286) reports, "Many investigators now believe that children who begin a depressed course before puberty are probably genetically driven into such an early expression of the illness." Impulsive children may have either bipolar illness, an attention deficit, or both. Some experts believe there are many more depressed children with this diagnosis than it was previously thought.

A Perspective on Childhood Depression

Two provocative quotes from Dr. Gold give both a perspective on depressive illness and a feeling for how children with the condition are often misunderstood.

He writes, "Depression in adults and children is remarkably alike...While the symptoms too are similar -- sleep and appetite disturbance, bodily complaints, hopelessness, guilt, lack of self-esteem, loss of ability to experience pleasure, fatigue and so on -- kids do not express them the same as grown-ups." As to the current lack of understanding and treatment of childhood depression, Gold (1987) states, "Many kids end up being treated for hyperactivity and learning disabilities, punished for laziness, or even placed in detention for aggressive, destructive behaviors, when depression is the primary problem."

ADOLESCENT DEPRESSION

Much of what was described as characteristic of childhood depression is also true of adolescent depression. Similarly, much of what is characteristic of adolescent depression is also applicable to childhood depression. The major difference is that often the more socially withdrawn child will become outgoing during the teen years, only to once again return to being withdrawn in adulthood. This brief section on adolescent depression describes issues especially troublesome in the teen years.

Anxiety and Alcohol/Drug Use

Chapter 5, "Anxiety and Suicide Prevention," gives extensive information on the role that high anxiety states play in increasing the risk of suicide for people with depression. It also addresses the dangers of using alcohol and/or drugs to self-treat anxiety. Parents, teachers and health professionals need to be aware that adolescents who are depressed and anxious frequently self-medicate their condition by using alcohol and/or street drugs.

Hormones

Another factor frequently found in adolescence is the interplay of hormones and depression. The blossoming of sexuality and the connection between hormone balances and mood makes the adolescent especially susceptible to depression. It is not within the scope of this book to fully describe the connection between how brain chemistry can affect hormones and, conversely, how hormones in other parts of the body can affect depressive symptoms. One just needs to look at the high rate of suicide attempts, especially by teenage girls, to get an appreciation for the interplay of changing hormone levels and depression. Or just think about what we are now learning about PMS (pre-menstrual syndrome). These emotional storms of adolescence are especially difficult for young persons suffering from dysthymia who are already battling low mood.

The role of hormones in depression is just beginning to be understood as playing a part in a wider picture of chemical imbalance. This quote from a recent publication summarizes how far we have come in recognizing the bigger picture:

"In the early days of research, scientists thought in terms of relatively simple models of chemical imbalance. Depression, for example, was thought to stem from an insufficiency of norepinephrine, one of many substances mediating the transmission of nerve impulses in the brain. Now, few experts talk about 'too much' or 'too little' of a single chemical. Instead, they believe mood disorders are the result of a complex interplay among a variety of chemicals, including neurotransmitters and hormones." (Goode, 1990, p. 55).

Disappointments in Love

Adolescence is also when kids fall in love for the first time. This makes them vulnerable to reactive depression, the mood disorder caused by a loss of some kind. I have frequently heard parents of a young person who committed suicide preface their description of what happened with the remark, "He had broken up with his girlfriend," or "She had broken up with her boyfriend."

Personality Factors

Psychiatrists have observed a number of personality characteristics that makes one especially vulnerable to depression. Dr. Gold (1987) writes, "Persons who are worriers and perfectionists are known to be vulnerable to depression. Extraordinarily dependent individuals as well as introverts are also at risk." Dr. Klerman's (1984) research on depressed persons conducted after their recovery from a depressive episode also gives a profile of the personality factors which make people especially vulnerable to mood disorders. He writes, "The depressed patient who emerges in this profile is introverted, lacking in self-confidence, unassertive, dependent, pessimistic, and self-perceived as inadequate." The teen years are notorious for causing one to be hypercritical. If the adolescent's personality has a number of those other characteristics in it already, he or she is vulnerable to a depressive episode.

A GOAL

The symptoms of depression in childhood and adolescence are not so mysterious once we see them as similar to, but not exactly like, those of adults. Once parents, teachers and health care professionals truly recognize depression as a biological condition rather than someone's fault, we can begin to tackle it as we would any other health problem.

One of the most exciting prospects in the treatment of bipolar illness (a highly biological condition) is early intervention with young people. Youngsters whose parents have the condition are at high risk of becoming bipolar themselves. There may be a way of helping them during some of the vulnerable years, age 10 - 25, the age of onset of the illness for young persons today.

Researchers have discovered that once people have a manic-depressive episode, they are more likely to have future episodes. Doctors use the term "kindling" to describe the tendency for further episodes to occur more readily even without the presence of any stress in the environment. Without some form of intervention, the average number of episodes people with bipolar illness are likely to experience is sixteen.

Stability, on the other hand, tends to beget more stability. To maintain the desired stability, early administration of lithium and either carbamazapine or depakote is used during childhood, adolescence and early adulthood. Lithium has a long history of producing stability. The seizure medications block kindling. Administration of these medicines may either prevent the occurrence of the illness, or reduce the number of episodes. Even if it fails to prevent the illness from occurring, the use of these medications by young persons with a high risk for bipolar illness may serve to protect them during those years. With the suicide rate for 15 - 19 year olds throughout the early 1990's at 18/100,000 for boys and bipolar patients at high risk for suicide, I personally welcome this type of preventive medicine.

The goal is to provide the most effective, least expensive treatment to the great number of young people who suffer. By treating the young we can provide a life-long benefit to them and their families. The next chapter describes what can be done.

What's To Be Done?

T he exciting news about depression is that most people can be helped. Two types of short term psychotherapies have <u>proven</u> to be effective. Sometimes these therapies can lift a depression without the use of medication, but the general consensus is that medication plus therapy gives the quickest and the best results for adults. Persons with genetically-based depression often need medication to treat their condition because it is caused by brain chemistry. The combination of chemical intervention and a psychotherapy which focuses on the behavioral manifestations of their illnesses works for at least 80% of adults suffering from depression.

Although moods do often lift on their own without the use of some type of intervention, it frequently takes six to nine months or sometimes as long as two years for the depression to lift. Medications, on the other hand, often work in a matter of weeks. Depression causes a lot of pain and can disrupt or destroy a life. Antidepressant medication is an effective, humane treatment which reduces unnecessary suffering. Some adults prefer not to use medication. Adult clients and their doctors need to work together to decide if they can work safely on the depression without the use of medication.

What about the use of prescription medications for adolescents with depression? Medications are important for some teens, and for those who benefit from them, they are a blessing. For some they can even be life-saving. Medications, like everything else, must be approached with caution. In a recent lecture by adolescent psychology specialist Dr. Harry Hoberman, he noted that although antidepressants have proven to be effective for adults and for children, the efficacy for adolescents is not clear. This does not mean there are no teens who benefit from antidepressants; it simply means there should be a judicious use of these medications for that age group.

Just exactly why antidepressants may not have the same record of success for adolescents is not yet known. It makes me wonder if this phenomena may not relate to how body chemistry interacts with brain chemistry. In the preceding chapter, the fact that brain chemistry can produce pain in various parts of the body was explained. Later, under the subheading "hormones," it was pointed out that the converse is also true; chemicals in the body can produce symptoms of depressed mood. I do not know how the interaction of body chemistry on brain chemistry affects boys and men, but these facts about females may be relevant to the role of hormones and depression and may be a clue as to why antidepressants may not work as well for adolescents. We know that:

1. *The incidence of depression is twice as high for women as for men.*

2. *The rate of attempted suicides for adolescent females is much higher than it is for males. There are approximately 40 - 50 attempts for every completed suicide for adolescent females.*

3. *Approximately 80 percent of women experience at least a mild case of post-partum depression.*

4. The phenomena of pre-menstrual syndrome involves many of the symptoms of depression.

5. Girls typically out-perform boys academically until the beginning of adolescence. Since there is a connection between depression and decreased ability to concentrate, hormonal changes that affect mood may be part of the cause of declined school performance.

Hormonal changes in adolescents may become identified as one of the reasons antidepressants have not yet been proven to show the same level of efficacy for teenagers as they have for children or adults.

It is also interesting to note that the course of life-long depressive illness in high level primates (monkeys and apes) is similar to that of humans. Scientists have observed these animals in their natural habitat and found that depressed young primates are socially withdrawn during childhood, more socially outgoing as adolescents and then return to withdrawal during adulthood. Can these findings give hints to the biological reasons why antidepressant may not have the same efficacy for adolescents as they do for children and adults?

With this question in mind, it becomes evident that non-medication techniques that have proven helpful for people with depression need to be the key component in a program to help depressed young people. The National Institute of Mental Health sponsored a collaborative study on the treatment of depression. They studied the effectiveness of two different psychotherapies: cognitive therapy and interpersonal therapy. Both were found to be effective for mood disorders. Cognitive therapy focuses on the thinking errors made by the depressed people. During therapy, patients develop an awareness of the illogical nature of some of their assumptions, are guided to formulate more logical statements about the circumstances in their lives, and are taught to apply reasonable solutions to their problems. Cognitive therapy does not dwell on what happened to them in the past; it focuses on the here and now. Cognitive therapy is compatible with a classroom setting because the clients' work involves writing and homework.

The second effective treatment for depression focuses on the problems the patient is currently having with interpersonal relationships. The work involves developing social competency with people in their lives right now, such as spouses, friends, family members, colleagues, neighbors, and other social contacts.

One of the most cost-effective methods of helping young people with mild to severe depression is to offer a psychology class which teaches the basics of cognitive and interpersonal therapy. Cognitive therapy teaches logic as it applies to one's personal life. Interpersonal therapy teaches social competency. A class focusing on, personal logic and interpersonal skills would easily fit into the curriculum of a psychology class. This class would be useful to anyone with a mild to severe case of depression, as well as anyone interested in personal growth. The class could be offered as a social studies elective in any junior high, senior high, college, or technical school. Since depression affects the ability of a student to concentrate, a class such as this has the potential to generally assist the student academically. It more than justifies its existence as an important element in the academic curriculum of any school.

To understand what would be taught in a class like this, and to comprehend the ways depression manifests itself in illogical thinking and social problems, a description of these therapies is helpful. As the thinking errors found in depression are described, you will come to see just how common mild forms of depression are in our society today, and how the huge population of young people with mild cases of depression would benefit from a class in personal logic and interpersonal skills.

COGNITIVE THERAPY

Depressed people do not perceive what is happening in their environment accurately, and they do not think logically. One could say their thinking is distorted. Depressed individuals are not crazy; they just are not as logical as they could be. For example, hopelessness and helplessness result from the lack of clear perception of a life situation. Illogical conclusions are made and few options seem apparent. Cognitive therapy's focus on thinking errors is a straight-forward psychotherapy for depression, since it works directly with the problems people have. It teaches people to think more logically; in other words, to think straight.

Cognitive therapy was pioneered by Dr. Aaron Beck. It deals with pervasive negativity of thought patterns, identifies gross distortions in a patient's thinking, and allows people to be more objective and realistic. Dr. Beck identified ten common thinking errors depressed persons make. A colleague, Dr. David Burns (1980), describes these in his book Feeling Good. A brief summary of these common distortions in personal logic gives a picture of depressed thinking.

1. All-or-Nothing Thinking

This describes thinking of yourself in black-or-white terms. Depressed people think they are supposed to be absolutely perfect at all times. We are human, less than perfect. Depression causes self-critical thinking. Any mistake or any imperfection causes depressed persons to think they are a complete loser. This illogical perfectionism is the reason straight-A students feel like a failure just for getting one B on a test. When you expect to be perfect at all times, you fear any kind of mistake. The exaggerated expectation of all-or-nothing thinking sets people up for impossible demands and feelings of inadequacy and worthlessness for just being human.

2. Overgeneralization

Overgeneralization causes depressed people to think that something negative that happened in the past will happen again and again. The emotional pain depressed people feel from rejection is often caused by overgeneralization. An assumption is made that since one person rejected you, all people will respond in exactly the same way. There is no evidence for this assumption and it is illogical, but when depressed persons overgeneralize, they think that since there was one negative experience, there will always be negative reactions from people.

3. Mental Filter

This refers to the tendency to focus on a negative detail of a situation and then dwell on it. Exclusively focusing on a negative detail causes depressed people to think the whole situation is bad. Dr. Burns writes that it is as if depressed people are wearing a pair of eyeglasses that filters out all the good things in life and allows only the negative to be viewed. They do not know that what they see is distorted. They only know that what they perceive consists totally of negative experiences.

4. Disqualifying the Positive

Even more tragic is the distortion of translating a totally neutral or even potentially good experience into something negative. Depressed people with this thinking error do not ignore positive experiences; they distort them. An appreciation for this cognitive problem gives insight into why people will feel so badly even when wonderful things are happening to them. In the midst of outer circumstances that are positive, the lives of depressed people become a nightmare where everything is awful. They think of themselves as losers, worthless pieces of humanity. If the depression is less severe, disqualifying the positive may take the form of thinking of themselves as second-rate. This error in logic and perception is probably one of the most destructive distortions, because people maintain negative beliefs about themselves in the face of objective evidence to the contrary.

5. Jumping to Conclusions

Rather than being logical, depressed persons leap to conclusions that are not warranted by evidence. Dr. Burns gives two examples of this:

Mind reading: Depressed people assume others have the same low opinion of them that they have of themselves. Convinced of their own worthlessness,. they never confirm this conclusion with facts. The scientific method of checking an hypothesis (to discover the truth) would help to correct this error in logic.

The Fortune Teller Error: As they think of the future, depressed people jump to the conclusion that something terrible is going to happen. Predictions of coming disaster fit into their thinking even when they are unrealistic.

6. Magnification and Minimization

With magnification, any small error or challenge can become an overwhelmingly difficult problem. This distortion has sometimes been called catastrophizing because it can transform a fairly typical negative situation into a catastrophe. With minimization, any strength, any talent, or any good fortune is seen as something very small and insignificant. Depressed people combine these two distortions by magnifying their imperfections and minimizing their assets, a process that will always create a perception of being at best second rate and at worst a complete loser.

7. Emotional Reasoning

If people use their emotions as proof of their assumptions, the conclusion depressed people draw will be negative. One of the examples Dr. Burns gave of this form of logic was 'I feel like a dud, therefore I am a dud.' Moods reflect what we think and what we believe. If our thinking is distorted, our moods are distorted. Taking the negative moods as proof that we are bad or useless has no basis. Many depressed persons feel very guilty. Using emotional reasoning, they use the negative emotion of guilt as their proof that they must have done something bad. Other examples Dr. Burns cited are feelings of being overwhelmed as proof their problems are impossible resolve, feelings of inadequacy as proof they are worthless, low mood as proof they should do nothing. A secondary effect of this form of distortion is procrastination.

8. "Should" Statements

Depression can cause low energy. Depressed people may try to get themselves going by using "should" statements like, 'I should do this' or 'I should do that.' Any statement that tries to force or shame them into doing something causes an artificial pressure and creates resentment. Instead of motivating them to do something, it has the opposite effect by making them feel apathetic. These statements turn up the emotional stress. Setting a standard for themselves with statements of what they must or should do and then falling short of this artificial standard adds to their self-loathing.

9. Labeling and Mislabeling

This refers to the process by which they create a totally negative self-concept that is based on thinking errors. It is overgeneralization in its extreme form. Labeling themselves as a loser, as worthless, as a hopeless case is both simplistic and inaccurate. It is done from feelings of inadequacy, rather than from genuine insight.

10. Personalization

This distortion causes people to take responsibility for something when there is no basis in fact for them to do so. Depressed people draw the conclusion that what happened was their fault or in some way is a reflection of their inadequacy. Personalization causes unnecessary, uncalled-for guilt. Their sense of guilt is burdensome to the point of being crippling. Feeling that what others do is their responsibility means the weight of the world is on their shoulders.

Implications and Application of Cognitive Therapy

These ten cognitive errors or distortions are common in our time. If these thinking patterns are familiar to you, you can now see why some scientists believe depression to be epidemic during the 1970's, 80's and 90's. If you feel overwhelmed just reading the list, you understand how depressed people feel.

Dr. Beck's therapy helps patients take an aggressive approach with their illogical thoughts. He emphasizes self help by outlining a three-step program to help patients deal with these distortions. Patients actively work during the session and do homework during the eight to twelve weeks of therapy. The three-step system consists of:

1. *Training themselves to both recognize and record in writing the self-critical thoughts as they occur.*

2. *Labeling these thoughts as distortions.*

3. *Talking back to these distortions by presenting a more realistic self-evaluation of the situation. (Burns, 1980)*

In addition to the work in changing thinking patterns, Beck's cognitive therapy works to change depressed people's pattern of doing nothing -- a result of their feeling helpless. Taking positive action can make a substantial change in the way they feel. Cognitive therapy is a multifaceted approach with proven results. It is a non-medication program which not only reduces the pain of a depressive episode but often helps to prevent future occurrences of the condition. It has great potential of helping groups of adolescents and young adults deal with mild to severe cases of depression.

INTERPERSONAL THERAPY (IPT)

Cognitive therapy is not the only short term, focused psychotherapy with proven efficacy. The other is the interpersonal therapy described by Dr. Gerald Klerman. It is designed specifically for the treatment of depression, and like cognitive therapy, it was investigated as part of the large scale, multi-site research project known as the NIMH Collaborative Study of Psychotherapy of Depression. IPT's effectiveness is well established. Like cognitive therapy, IPT focuses on some of the specific symptoms of depression.

An analysis of the list of symptoms of mood disorders reveals a cluster of issues revolving around the problems people have getting along with others. Children, adolescents, and adults with depression often are angry and irritable, dependent, fearful, unable to experience pleasure, socially isolated, or withdrawn. They suffer from low self-esteem and low energy. Depressed people with those symptoms may not be anyone's first choice for a friend. The interpersonal aspects of depression consequently are as fruitful an avenue for work as are the cognitive distortions.

The basic premise of Dr. Klerman's IPT is that depression occurs within an interpersonal context. He believes that intervention and training which focus on the interpersonal context helps people recover from a mild or severe depression and may even help to prevent future depression. Klerman's focused, short-term program emphasizes the patient's specific problems with current interpersonal relations. Although there is full recognition of the importance genetics and brain chemistry have in predisposing the individual to depression and an understanding that personal history and personality factors also play an important role in causing vulnerability to depression, IPT focuses on how to deal with the social problems resulting from the depressive condition. There is no in-depth analysis of the past or any attempt to change basic personality. IPT focuses instead on "current disputes, frustrations, anxieties, and wishes as defined in the interpersonal context." (Klerman, 1984, p. 7).

Dr. Klerman's approach relies on well-established techniques such as:

1. *reassurance,*
2. *clarification of emotional states,*
3. *improvement of interpersonal communication,*
4. *testing of perceptions and performance through interpersonal contact.*

IPT is a no-fault approach to teaching social skills. The fact that young people with depression lack interpersonal skills is not their fault. The significant people in their lives (their parents, teachers, friends) may not be at fault either. Past and current interpersonal problems are related to the depression, but they are not necessarily anyone's fault. Klerman reminds us that persons with serious depression may:

Exaggerate and distort problems in their interpersonal relations because of their current affective state and cognitive dysfunction. The symptoms of the depression.... and the patient's personality may make the people less competent to establish mutually satisfying interpersonal relationships and maintain attachments. (Klerman, 1984)

A no-fault approach to teaching social skills is not only therapeutic, it also fits the facts. For example, any blame affixed to parents for creating the depression in a young person with a genetically driven illness like bipolar or unipolar recurrent depression cannot be supported by current research findings that do not associate the depression with low maternal care or overprotection. (Klerman, 1984). Nor is it the teacher's fault either that some students' low energy, low self-esteem, and feelings of helplessness and hopelessness may lead them to disinterest in school work. It is not the peers' fault that the anger and irritability symptoms of some types of depression makes some classmates difficult to get along with. Mostly, it is not depressed people's fault they have these symptoms. IPT, through its work with reassurance,   clarification of emotional state, improvement in communications, and testing of perceptions and performance through interpersonal contact, improves social skills and relieves depression.   It has a rightful place in the curriculum of a psychology class which can be made available in our schools.

COGNITIVE THERAPY AND IPT: A USEFUL CLASS FOR HELPING TODAY'S PROBLEMS

When describing the use of cognitive and IPT techniques (and in select cases, antidepressant medication) for the almost 40% of our population who are mildly to severely depressed, an analogy with orthodontia is useful. Many people are blessed with reasonably straight teeth and do not need braces. However, quite a sizable portion of the population do have crooked teeth. Good old Mother Nature gave them a problematic bite. It is not their fault their teeth are crooked. The teeth are not crooked because they were too weak-willed to have them come in straight. No amount of determination on their part is going to make those teeth straighten up. The same is true for people with depression. Many lucky people never experience the pain of depression, but quite a sizable portion of our population do. Through no fault of their own, they too need outside assistance.

If a person with a troublesome bite wants to go through life with straight teeth, he will have to do something about it. Sometimes an oral surgeon needs to pull out teeth to make room in the mouth before efforts are made to straighten the remaining teeth. Some people do not need to have teeth pulled; braces alone will work, but for a sizable percentage of the people needing orthodontia, teeth have to come out if the braces are going to be successful. The same is true for depression. For many adults with depression, medication is the first step in getting the help they need. Only after three to six weeks on medication will cognitive and IPT therapy be fruitful.

When orthodontists put on braces, they put pressure on those teeth to move them into a different pattern. Similarly, the cognitive therapist and the client work aggressively on illogical thoughts and overly critical perceptions. They take them in hand, getting tough with distorted logic to straighten up. This type of therapy allows people to be more objective and positive in their thinking, and ultimately begin to treat themselves more kindly. They are tough on their thinking, but good to themselves.

Once the braces are off, people often wear a retainer to keep those beautifully straightened teeth in line, so problems will not recur. Likewise, some continuing but less intense work on cognitive training can be done by the patients themselves or in support groups to retain the benefits of the new thinking patterns.

Just because you may come from a family in which there is a genetic predisposition to having a crowded bite, it does not mean you necessarily have to go through life with an unattractive smile or dental problems. Something can be done about it. It may cost some money and take some time, but the odds are you will have a very satisfactory result. The same is generally true for depressive illness. You may come from a family with a genetic predisposition to depressive illness, but there is something that you can do about it. It may cost some money and take some time, but the odds are you will have satisfactory results.

Orthodontia can be done at any age. People in their 30's, 40's and 50's can and do wear braces. But generally, braces are worn by people in their teens and twenties. We believe the problem might as well be dealt with when it first becomes apparent. Resolving the problem when the person is young gives a lifetime worth of benefit from the braces. Furthermore, since crowded teeth are harder to care for, people with a problematic bite can develop a mouthful of cavities as well.

The same is true of depression. Although some people have their first depressive episode in their 30's, 40's, 50's or beyond, today we are seeing first depressive episodes in children, teens, and people in their twenties. Parents, teachers, and doctors who recognize the symptoms of depression will want to deal with it when it first becomes apparent so that individual can have a lifetime worth of benefit from effective treatment. Furthermore, like the mouth full of cavities that people may develop, the individual with depressive illness may develop additional problems like alcohol and/or drug abuse, impaired personal relationships, problems with work, etc., that might have been avoided if they had gotten treatment when the symptoms first appeared.

I hope to see the day when the practice of mental health becomes similar to the practices of dentistry. In order for that to happen, the general public has the right to demand evidence that the money spent on helping themselves or their family members will be well spent. We all have the right to expect that the methods used have proven efficacy. If schools include an elective class using cognitive therapy and IPT, they will be using methods with proven effectiveness. It is a cost-effective means of helping the nearly 40% of our school population with mild to severe depression gain the skills they need. It will give them a lifetime of benefit.

There is one important distinction between having crooked teeth and having a genetically driven depression like bipolar and unipolar recurrent depression. Having crooked teeth will not kill you. Depression might.

Anxiety and
Suicide Prevention

I f we hope to help young people at risk for committing suicide, we need to not only understand depression, but anxiety. Anxiety is a very different problem. Symptoms of anxiety can foretell who is at imminent risk for making a serious attempt or actually completing suicide.

What is anxiety? It is fearfulness in the absence of an environmental reason for fear. For example, if a child is called into the principal's office he is likely to perceive a problem and will have a reason to feel frightened. If, on the other hand, a child with average or above average academic skills feels frightened every time he enters the classroom, that is anxiety.

The symptoms of general anxiety disorder are:

A. Excessive anxiety and worry (apprehensive expectation), occurring more days than not for at least 6 months, about a number of events or activities (such as work or school performance).

B. The person finds it difficult to control the worry.

C. The anxiety and worry are associated with three (or more) of the following six symptoms (with at least some symptoms present for more days than not for the past 6 months). **Note**: Only one item is required in children.

1. *restlessness or feeling keyed up or on edge*
2. *being easily fatigued*
3. *difficulty concentrating or mind going blank*
4. *irritability*
5. *muscle tension*
6. *sleep disturbance (difficulty falling or staying asleep, or restless unsatisfying sleep (DSM-IV)*

Persons with high anxiety are prone to panic attacks. The prevalence of panic attacks was researched by Dr. Myrna Weissman (1991) as part of the Epidemiologic Catchment Area Study funded by the National Institute of Mental Health. About four percent of persons interviewed by Weissman's study had experienced such attacks. During an attack, the person had the symptoms of high anxiety, as well as experiencing: dizziness, hot and cold flashes, fainting, trembling, and a fear of dying or going crazy. As compared to the chronic state of anxiety the person usually feels, a panic attack is an acute, time-limited state of intense anxiety which produces a feel of impending doom.

Panic attacks are recurring episodes that come upon the person suddenly and unpredictably. These attacks of fear can be crippling. Persons with anxiety disorder sometimes are frightened to be alone. Not knowing when the next crippling attack might occur, panic sufferers often want the support of someone near at hand. It is also common for persons with anxiety disorder to fear public places away from home because after several attacks, they will avoid places that resemble those where episodes of panic occurred in the past. In extreme cases, the fear of having another attack will cause them to become immobile. Dr. Weissman reports that approximately 1.5% of the population have panic attacks some time in their lives that are severe or prolonged enough to be diagnosed as Panic Disorder.

Anxiety disorders are common for people with depressive illness. The term dysphoria means the combination of depression and anxiety so often seen by psychiatrists. Dr. Gerald Klerman (1984, p. 31) observed that "approximately 60 to 70 percent of depressed patients report anxiety." This was true for my son Ben. As a child he was frightened in situations in which there were no environmental reasons to feel fear. He was uncomfortable being alone or sleeping alone. We tried to encourage him to be more independent, but many nights it was kinder to allow him to fall asleep in our bed and then move him to his own once he was asleep. A picture of Ben when he was eighteen months old showed him biting his nails. This photo is helpful to me in appreciating the long-term nature of his experience with the symptoms of his anxiety disorder and the biological nature of the condition.

When he became school aged, he went to school each day, but it was not a comfortable situation for him. Unlike most young boys who are out playing with friends, Ben chose to be at home with us or with a very few other people who allowed him to feel less anxious. If he went away from home to play, he always wanted either my husband or me to go with him.

Another anxiety symptom Ben experienced was dizziness. There were times when Ben fell while walking down a short flight of stairs. He would explain that he fell because he was dizzy. His dizziness did not make any sense to me at the time, but it is indicative of his anxiety disorder.

The summer following Ben's sixth grade, I observed what I now know was a panic attack. On a camping trip Ben told me his heart was beating fast and he was frightened. His heart would not slow down, and he said he felt like he was having a heart attack. I had him lie down and do some deep breathing to help him relax until it passed. I do not recall how long the attack lasted. He rested for some time and later reported the palpitations stopped. It was a very painful experience for him to have and for me to watch. It seems a shame that a child this young should have to experience something so frightening.

Although many people have an anxiety disorder which accompanies their depressive condition, anxiety can occur alone. Suicide attempts are made by persons who experience panic attacks without the concurrent depression. Dr. Weissman (1991) discovered that "the lifetime rate of suicide attempts in persons with uncomplicated Panic Disorder (without any other problem such as depression) was seven percent, consistently higher than the one percent rate for persons with no psychiatric disorder." What is more, Dr. Weissman's research unexpectedly discovered that for all panic patients (those with anxiety disorders occurring along with other problems such as depression, as well as those with anxiety alone), the rate of suicide attempts rose to 20 percent. She writes, "Therefore, we concluded that suicide attempts were associated with Panic Disorder in its uncomplicated, or its comorbid form, and the risks were comparable to those of major depression, both comorbid and uncomplicated." These findings were substantiated by similar findings both in Europe and in Canada. They underscore the importance of treating panic attacks as one way of reducing the risk of suicide attempts.

Furthermore, clinicians want to know which of their patients are acutely suicidal and which patients have symptoms that indicate a chronic state of high suicide risk. Eminent psychiatrist Dr. Jan Fawcett analyzed the symptoms "which would discriminate highly suicidal patients from the majority of depressed patients who do not kill themselves." His preliminary findings indicate the important role anxiety plays as a risk factor.

As part of the Collaborative Program on the Psychobiology of Depression, Fawcett (1992) analyzed the one year follow-up data of 954 patients with severe depression. He found six variables "are significantly related to suicide within one year of entry into the study." These variables are:

   1. panic attack
   2. severe psychic anxiety
   3. diminished concentration
   4. global insomnia
   5. moderate alcohol abuse
   6. severe loss of interest or pleasure (anhedonia).

Variables that are reliable long-term predictors of suicide occurring sometime in the patients' future are:

   1. hopelessness
   2. suicidal ideation
   3. previous suicidal attempts. (Fawcett, 1992, p. 104)

The importance of paying serious attention to the role high anxiety states can have on suicide attempts or completion was discussed in an interview Dr. Fawcett gave for the newsletter "Livesaver," published by the American Suicide Foundation (1991, Summer). When asked why panic attacks can prove to be deadly, his response was, "When panic attacks occur together with the hopelessness that can accompany depression, patients may begin to feel that only suicide can provide some relief. It is easy to see how someone in that situation could feel desperate and hopeless, anticipating the pain of severe panic attacks that will continue to recur." Fawcett went on to recommend educating people about the existence of Panic Disorder as a treatable condition.

The co-existence of panic attacks in persons with depression increases the risk of suicide. This is evident from the fact that "in the study's first year 62 percent of the patients who killed themselves had panic attacks together with major depression." ("Understanding," 1991). Panic attacks usually occur in about 25 to 30 percent of clients who have a serious depressive illness. Anxiety is probably the most dangerous problem a person with depression can have.

What are the implications of these findings for physicians? Dr. Fawcett says, "Patients with a major affective disorder who have marked anxiety, panic attacks or agitation, should be recognized as imminent suicide risks by the treating clinicians." These patients need to be treated pharmacologically and with other appropriate measures.

The implication of the work of Drs. Weissmann and Fawcett leads to a conclusion that clients with high anxiety levels have a high risk for attempting suicide sometime in their lives; moreover, the presence of panic attacks in depressed persons places them at imminent risk of making suicide attempts.

NON-MEDICATION
TREATMENT FOR ANXIETY
WITH OR WITHOUT DEPRESSION

What about the many young people whose anxiety interferes with effective functioning? Medication is often a necessary part of treatment for anxiety disorder, especially when it is severe or prolonged enough to meet the criteria for Panic Disorder and/or if the patient is seriously depressed.

There may be two type of anxiety disorders. In the first type, much that can be said about depression is also true of that type of anxiety, and it responds to the same medication -- antidepressants. The other type of anxiety disorder does not respond to antidepressants. What are the other treatments for anxiety besides medications? Are there any inexpensive means of helping young people to manage their anxiety?

In the previous chapter I suggested the development of a course that could be offered to any adolescent. It treated the major symptoms of depression: the cognitive errors and problems with interpersonal relationships. The curriculum of this class should also include elements that help young people manage their anxiety. It could include the following five items.

1. Information on the biological nature of anxiety.

Anxiety, like depression, is probably a result of biological predispositions. Anxiety disorders, like many other conditions, tend to run in families. Persons who have "a close relative with the condition were more likely to develop it than those who did not." (Sheehan, 1983). Studies suggest that "proneness to this disorder fit closely, though not perfectly, with a dominant-gene inheritance pattern." (Sheehan, 1983, p. 82). In this type of pattern, a person could inherit the disorder from just one parent.

The biological nature of the condition is also reflected in its strong association with a heart condition called mitral valve prolapse.

Among patients with panic attacks, approximately one in every three also has this disorder, which involves a floppy mitral valve in the heart. This floppy mitral valve is believed to be inherited through a dominant gene. The disorder is not usually considered a serious heart problem. Although no one yet fully understands the relationship between the two conditions, the frequent coexistence of the anxiety disease with the inherited mitral valve prolapse lends some further support to the idea that there is some genetic vulnerability to the anxiety disease. (Sheehan, 1983, pp. 82-83)

Studying characteristics of twins lends further credence to the genetic inheritability of anxiety disease. Twin studies are used to separate behavior resulting from the effects of environment versus behavior due to the effects of heredity. When identical twins are compared with non-identical twins in regard to anxiety disorders, heredity appears to be of greater importance than environment. The scientific community is now trying to discover the exact biochemical or metabolic abnormality that causes this condition.

> The best guesses so far involve certain nerve endings and receptors in the central nervous system which produce and receive chemical messengers that stimulate and excite the stimulants called catecholamines. It is believed that in the anxiety disease, the nerve endings are overfiring. They are working too hard, overproducing these stimulants and perhaps others.
>
> At the same time there are nerve endings and receptors that have the opposite effect: they produce naturally-occurring tranquilizers, called inhibitory neurotransmitters, that inhibit, calm down, and dampen the nerved firing of the brain. It appears that the neurotransmitters or the receptors may be deficient, either in quality or quantity. (Sheehan, 1983, pp. 83-84)

Learning these facts and others relative to the biological nature of this condition is cognitively therapeutic. Persons with any illness need some reassurance that their problems are not their fault. People with anxiety disorders especially need to know their condition is a treatable medical illness. It is not a hopeless condition and they are not helpless because it exists. Like any other medical problem, it must be managed by the person who has it. Developing self-help skills is a must.

2. Teaching Breathing Techniques

Several symptoms of high anxiety states and panic attacks involve breathing: e.g., difficulty in getting breath or overbreathing, smothering or choking sensations or lump in throat, dizziness, and fainting. If we are to help people with anxiety, we must help them feel that they have more control over their breathing. When recommending a technique, I always feel more confident turning to an ancient method -- one that has withstood the test of time. Here is what eminent teacher and author Joseph Campbell (1990) says about Kundalini yoga:

"The notion is that emotion and feeling and state of the mind are related to breath. When you are at rest, the breathing is in a nice, even order. When you are stirred with shock the breathing changes. With passion the breathing changes. Change the breathing and you change the state."

Routinely practicing yoga could be a means of decreasing part of the symptoms associated with high anxiety states. This book cannot go into great detail about yoga techniques, but Campbell gives this simple summary of how yoga is practiced. One starts with controlling the breath by means of specific breathing paces. "You breathe in through one nostril, hold, breathe out through the other nostril, hold in through the second, hold, out through the first and so forth and so on." (Campbell, 1990, p. 136).

Picture in your mind a person doing yoga, and then a person experiencing a high anxiety state. Aren't those incompatible images? Wouldn't it be advisable to use this well-established practice to help people with anxiety disorder? Yoga may provide to be a method of breath training that would reduce one of the major symptoms of high anxiety states.

3. Teaching the Use of Visualization

Visualization is useful in both raising self concept and in decreasing anxiety. The book Self-Esteem, by Matthew McKay and Patrick Fanning, describes the technique and how it works. Visualization work starts first with teaching the person to relax, to clear the mind of distractions, and to imagine positive peaceful scenes. In this calm state, students imagine themselves doing things successfully, such as interacting pleasantly with others or achieving goals easily, etc.

Visualization works to reduce the fear component of anxiety. As stated earlier, anxiety is defined as fearfulness in the absence of any environmental reasons for feeling frightened. This is how visualization works: In the relaxation phase, the instructor guides students through a process that allows them to relax every part of their body. Once relaxed, they are instructed to calmly focus on improving their ability to experience each of their senses. Students visualize a vivid scene: details of what the scene looks like, the sounds they might hear, the tactile experience they will have, what might be tasted or eaten in the place, and the smell they would encounter. As students practice forming these sensory images, they become better at doing visualization.

Once they have improved their ability to visualize, students may want to identify situations that frighten them or identify desired goals in everyday life that are blocked by anxiety states. Using visualization techniques allows them to imagine scenes in which they are calm and able to perform in a relaxed, confident manner. They imagine themselves doing what they want to do easily. Students are encouraged to practice visualization techniques at home, especially at night before falling asleep and in the morning after awakening. These are times when they are naturally in a relaxed state. This is especially helpful for the "difficulty falling asleep" symptom characteristic of anxiety and the "global insomnia" symptom associated with a high risk of suicide. It gives individuals an opportunity to use the time spent in bed when they are unable to sleep. The relaxation step of visualization may actually help them to fall asleep. But even if they do not sleep, they will feel relaxed while concentrating on scenes in which they are calm, successful, and happy.

4. Teaching the Use of Affirmations

Affirmations work like visualizations, but they are verbal statements rather than images. The author of <u>Creative Visualization</u>, Shakti Gawain (1978) writes "An affirmation is a strong, positive statement that something is <u>already</u> so. It is a way of making firm that which you are imaging."

Gawain's book gives a number of examples of affirmations that would be helpful to persons with anxiety:

1. Everything is coming to me easily and effortlessly.
2. Everything I need is already within me.
3. I love and appreciate myself just as I am.

4. I am whole and complete in myself.

5. I am always in the right place at the right time,
   successfully engaged in the right activity.

6. It's okay for me to have fun and enjoy myself and I
   do.

7. I am relaxed and centered - I have plenty of time
   for everything.

8. I now enjoy everything I do.

                        (Gawain, 1978, pp. 22-23)

Gawain gives many other examples of affirmations for a wide variety of potentially stressful situations. It could be performance anxiety in academics, sports, work, financial difficulties, or stress arising from difficulties in interpersonal relations. Students can even be encouraged to write an affirmation of their own concerning problems they want resolved in their lives.

The particular strength of affirmations is that students are able to use them at times when it is impossible to use other techniques. You do not have to put yourself in a state of relaxation in order to use affirmations. You can just say these statements any time you need to (e.g., right before a test) or any time you want to (e.g., while waiting for a bus).

Personally, I find writing affirmations to be helpful. The process of moving my hand and seeing the words on the page has a powerful effect. It helps me to concentrate, something we all find hard to do when we are anxious. I can write two or three affirmations over and over again while I am stuck somewhere waiting, and it gives me something positive to do. The calming effect of doing this simple repetitive act with its potential for a positive outcome by itself reduces the anxiety that can arise in the course of everyday life.

Two of the three long-term predictors of suicide are hopelessness and suicidal ideation (frequent thoughts of committing suicide) . What better way to combat hopelessness than by strong, positive statements? What better way to combat intrusive ideas about killing yourself than by writing affirmations (firm statements) about positive things happening in your life?

5. Teaching that alcohol and drug abuse is an ineffective means of self-treating anxiety

Today's parents are frightened their teenagers may begin to experiment with drugs and alcohol. What they may not see is that this behavior is often an attempt to self-treat anxiety. Adolescents who have both depression and anxiety may not be able to accidentally discover a treatment for the depression but will discover that alcohol relieves anxiety. I wish to emphasize that although alcohol does reduce the symptoms of anxiety, it is itself a depressive drug -- it makes the depression worse. If depressed and anxious adolescent and young adults self-medicate with alcohol, they will end up trading reduced anxiety now for greater depression later. Because alcohol gives people an immediate and temporary lift it is hard to convince depressed adolescents that they are actually making the depression worse. Their solution to any new low is to get high again. Others may recognize the self-destructive nature of their behavior, but persons who abuse alcohol and drugs may only see that they are getting some relief from discomfort.

I hope I will not be misunderstood. I realize not everyone who abuses alcohol or becomes addicted to drugs does so because they are anxious and/or depressed people who self-medicate their condition. Researchers alert us to the number of previously not depressed people who develop depression as a result of abusing alcohol and other depressive drugs. It is important to make a distinction between people with an underlying depression and/or anxiety disorder versus people who become depressed from using and abusing drugs. We must be careful to treat these two groups differently. Severely anxious and depressed adolescents may need antidepressant medication, but the abusive person may simply need to stop taking the drugs.

Furthermore, mental health professionals now distinguish two types of alcoholism. Adolescent onset patients have this condition before age 20. It is highly genetic. These alcoholics have differences in their serotonin levels and do not respond as well to the 12-step program. Adult onset patients develop their illness after age 20. This condition is an interplay of both genetic predisposition and abusive behavior. They respond well to the 12-step program. Alcoholics Anonymous still is the most effective treatment for these clients.

An important part of any class to help young people today should include a component about alcohol and drugs. The difficulty lies in finding an approach that will have an effect on behavior. While I don't know of any approach that has proven to be successful, perhaps you do. Or maybe your school system is already using one that is helpful. There are indications that the use of street drugs has declined with efforts to tell the whole truth about their negative effects. Similarly, efforts to change the image of drug use from one of glamour, adventure, and fun, to a more accurate image of increased dependency and depression, are also helpful. Educators know that teaching methods which engage students in discussion rather than passively receiving information produces a greater impact on behavior. Methods that combine all these approaches would likely have some success.

THE USE OF PRESCRIPTION DRUGS FOR ANXIETY

The antidepressants used to treat the type of anxiety that responds to medicine are the MAO inhibitors and the SSRIs. The following chapter on medications describes these in detail.

It was stated earlier that although antidepressants are proving to be effective for adults, their efficacy for treatment of adolescent depression is not clear. Their efficacy for treatment of anxiety in adolescents is also unclear. Medications for teens may be helpful (perhaps especially when panic attacks are frequent), but they need to be used cautiously with this age group. Like the treatment of depression, non-medication methods need to be the key component in a program to help young people cope with anxiety.

Offering an elective class to any interested student would provide an inexpensive way of treating mild to moderate forms of anxiety. It would also augment the therapy and/or medication that a specialist would provide for someone who has a serious problem with this disorder. A course that actually provides treatment is a very different approach from what has been done in the past. Hotlines have not worked. (Someone who is serious about attempting suicide is more likely to reach for a bottle of pills or a gun than a telephone.) Educational programs that only increase awareness have not worked. Giving information does

not necessarily translate into changed behavior the w
training does. Providing information on how to obtain he
not translate into people actually going out to seek help when
they need it.

Actual treatment that is easily accessible and affordable is
essential. An elective class that provides treatment for two
clusters of symptoms of depression, the distorted thinking
(cognitive therapy), and the problems with everyday relationships
(interpersonal skills training), as well as treatment for anxiety
(described by the five non-medication techniques in this chapter)
has real potential to help young people.

I recognize not everyone who commits suicide is
depressed or anxious, but these two conditions are associated
with the majority of these deaths. Those who wish to work
toward suicide prevention are putting their efforts today into
increasing the number of persons getting treatment for these
conditions. Using proven methods and techniques that have a
high likelihood of reducing anxiety and depression, and
formulating a curriculum for an elective class offer the best hope
for treating large numbers of young people today. Burns' Ten
Days to Self-Esteem is the kind of text that has already *proven* to
be effective for groups of depressed young people.

THE ROLE OF MEDICATION

I used to think that doctors discovered the nature of an illness and then chemists designed a medicine to treat it. I have since learned that often medical discoveries are like any other discovery; they are lucky accidents. Sometimes after a substance is found which reduces the symptoms of an illness, scientists will then set out to learn how the medicine works. During this process they begin to learn more about the nature of the illness itself. For example, the early effective medications for depression were discovered between 1949 and 1956. But it is only in recent years that scientists are beginning to unravel the mystery behind these conditions.

LITHIUM:
The Story Behind the Discovery

Lithium helps to stabilize persons by reducing the severity of future recurrences of both the manic and depressive phases of bipolar illness. The history of this medication is fascinating. As Dr. Fieve points out in his classic book, <u>Moodswings</u>, it was not a discovery at all but a rediscovery. We have actually had the treatment for the last 1800 years. Fieve writes:

> In the early Greek and Roman tent hospitals some eighteen hundred years ago, the physician Soramus of Ephesus prescribed mineral-water therapy for manic insanity and melancholia. In fact, he advocated in his writing the use of specific alkaline springs for a number of physical and mental illnesses. The tradition persisted for centuries. Today many of these alkaline springs developed by the Romans in southern and western Europe are known to contain high quantities of lithium. (p. 207-208)

Lithium is a perfectly natural substance found on the atomic chart right along with all the other basic elements, such as hydrogen and oxygen.

It gets its name from the Greek word for stone (lithos) because it is usually found in stone - mineral rock. It is also found in mineral waters and in some plant, animal, and human tissues. Historically, lithium has been used to treat a variety of conditions. Fieve writes that one century ago it was used to treat gout, rheumatism, and many other physical as well as mental diseases. Lithium salts, when added to uric acid had been used to dissolve kidney stones. I personally find the connection between rheumatism and lithium interesting. I know a number of persons with depression who also are plagued with arthritic pain, swelling, and crippling. One friend who now takes lithium for his bipolar illness has experienced significant improvement in his arthritis.

Additionally, there is a connection between the treatment of bipolar illness and the treatment of seizure disorder. In the first part of this century, lithium bromide was used to treat epilepsy. As more effective medications were developed to control seizures, the use of lithium for epilepsy was discontinued. Now the connection between treatment of epilepsy and bipolar illness is again emerging. Doctors today are finding that two medications developed for the treatment of epilepsy can be helpful to some persons with bipolar illness. These medicines, carbamazepine and valproic acid, are sometimes used by patients who do not tolerate lithium. Most often these medications are used in combination with lithium to produce greater stability in a patient's moodswings.

The story of lithium's specific use to control bipolar illness is a combination of both good luck and unfortunate coincidence. Fieve writes that in 1949 the Australian psychiatrist John F. Cade suspected the urea found in the urine of manic patients to be the toxin which created the manic state. To test his hypothesis he decided to inject guinea pigs with uric acid. He needed a soluble salt to add to this acid. When he injected the lithium urate into the guinea pigs they did not become manic as he had hypothesized. Instead they became lethargic. This also occurred when he injected the guinea pigs with lithium carbonate alone. Based on these findings, he then gave lithium carbonate to ten manic patients. They all experienced positive calming effects. Cade reported these findings.

The unfortunate coincidence which prevented the use of lithium from being of help to patients with bipolar illness also occurred in the late 1940s. In the United States, lithium chloride was being sold in stores as a salt substitute for persons who needed a sodium-free diet. Obviously, some of the persons who were buying lithium to season their food were people with heart and kidney disease. We now know that people who take lithium need to have salt (sodium chloride) in their diet in order to excrete lithium. Without sodium, the kidney conserves lithium and people can become lithium toxic, which is why these people died. When several deaths with these patients were reported in 1949, lithium was quickly taken off the market.

These deaths caused the American medical community to become extremely cautious about further use of lithium. It was the Danish psychiatrist Mogens Schou who began in 1954 to develop the use of lithium for the treatment of manic-depressive illness. In 1958 the use of lithium was studied in New York State and later in Texas. After more than a decade of study in the United States, it was finally approved by the FDA in 1970. As Dr. Fieve points out in his book, this is "twenty years after its discovery. " (p.211).

Proponents of lithium do not claim that it can prevent all future manic or depressive episodes or that there are no side effects. Bipolar illness is a serious condition and moodswings do still occur for many patients. Side effects such as hand tremors, nausea, and diarrhea are possible. However, many bipolar patients experience dramatic positive results from its use and regard lithium as a truly remarkable medicine for their condition. They and many others are grateful to Dr. Modes Schou for his pioneer work in proving that this medicine works.

Lithium for Young Patients

Psychiatrists estimate that anywhere from one-fourth to one-half of young people whose symptoms indicate depression are really suffering from bipolar illness. These children have symptoms you will recognize if you read Ben's Story. They include stomach aches, headaches, dizziness, bed-wetting, and difficulty concentrating on schoolwork. The children often are phobic. Parents and teachers report bursts of aggressiveness and frantic activity alternating with periods of sluggishness. Sometimes these children are helped during these early stages of their condition by the use of some kinds of antidepressants, since their first symptoms point to depression. When lithium is used with the antidepressants, the lithium appears to reduce the bodily complaints experienced by the children, and the antidepressant reduces their irritability. What happens during adolescence? Undiagnosed and untreated, these young people with bipolar illness are often described as having a behavioral disorder or a character disorder. Their impulsive pleasure seeking behavior alternates with sullen moods. They typically do not respond well to tricyclic antidepressants. But if the clients and the families are willing to give lithium enough time to produce its stabilizing effects, their response to lithium is often remarkable.

The Use of Lithium as a Maintenance Medicine for Bipolar Illness

If the person is not experiencing an acute problem with either mania or severe depression, lithium alone is sometimes used. But psychiatrists today are finding that many patients cannot remain stable with lithium alone. Like patients with epilepsy who often need two medications to prevent or decrease the number of seizures, bipolar clients often need both lithium and Depakene (valproic acid; divalproex) or lithium and Tegretol (carbamazepine) to prevent or reduce the severity of their moodswings. Furthermore, like some persons with epilepsy who require three medications to manage their seizures, some bipolar patients who are not stabilized by either lithium and Depakene or lithium and Tegretol are helped when lithium and Depakene and Tegretol are prescribed.

Use of Other Medications for Acute Episodes of Mania or Depression

Lithium, which helps to stabilize temperament by preventing future moodswings, usually does not work quickly enough to be useful during an acute attack. Bipolar patients who experience mania will need antipsychotic/neuroleptics medicines such as Mellaril, Thorazine, or Trilafon or many others. These medicines are discontinued by many patients soon after the manic episode subsides.

During a swing down into severe depression, bipolar patients will likely benefit from one of the four classes of anti-depressants: a tricyclic such as Tofranil (imipramine), a MAO inhibitor such as Nardil or Parnate, a SSRIs such as Prozac (fluoxetine), and the fourth type of antidepressant, Wellbutrin (bupropion). These medicines too will be discontinued for some patients with bipolar illness soon after the depressive symptoms subside.

Importance of Continuing Maintenance Medication for Bipolar Clients

There are several reasons why it is essential to continue lithium and/or Depakene or Tegretol as an ongoing treatment for bipolar illness. (Since lithium has become the most widely used medicine for decades in the treatment of this illness and is sometimes the only medicine needed to produce stability, I will refer only to lithium when describing why it is important not to discontinue using maintenance medication during periods of stability.)

Bipolar patients who stop lithium can become highly unstable, often more unstable than they were before starting the medicine.

This is not a negative statement indicating that lithium can cause this instability. It is more a reflection on how essential the medicine is for bipolar patients who need it.

Discontinuation of lithium can sometimes interfere with the ability of the person to benefit from the medicine once it is started again.

Some persons who have been stabilized (sometimes for years) on lithium decide for one reason or another to go off the medicine. Some of these people do not experience the same stability when they resume taking lithium as they had before. This phenomena is called "Withdrawal Induced Refractory," meaning that stopping the medication caused the person to become non-responsive to the medicine in the future. Although lithium typically takes time to become effective, and one does not expect to see restabilization for many months, some unfortunate persons who stop lithium can retake it again for years and still not have the same level of stability they had during the many years they took it the first time.

Lithium dramatically decreases the likelihood a bipolar patient will commit suicide.

Bipolar illness is a serious form of depression. The suicide rate among these patients is nearly 20 percent. When lithium is effective in preventing further episodes of moodswings, patients feel less helpless and less hopeless about their condition. It is not surprising that it can help to prevent suicide.

With these powerful reasons for staying on lithium, why would a bipolar client want to discontinue taking it? The reasons are:

1. *After stabilization, the person may begin to believe that they really do not have bipolar illness after all.*

2. *Some bipolar clients use the early stage of manic highs to do productive work.*

3. *Weight gain occurs for some patients.*

4. *Other side effects, such as interference with concentration or fatigue, trouble the client.*

The physicians who are most successful in helping bipolar clients always address these issues. For example, the problems with concentration, memory, and fatigue can be reduced by:

1. *taking all of the lithium at bedtime rather than throughout the day,*

2. *keeping the thyroid level in the high normal range by taking synthroid if necessary,*

3. *taking folic acid either by itself or as part of a multiple vitamin.*

Clients need support if they are to stay on lithium. This can come from family and friends, but an important addition to this is a manic-depressive support group. Whatever the source of support, persons with bipolar illness need to confront the effect that their illness can have on themselves and their family. They also need support in a daily regimen that includes exercise, a healthy diet and good sleep habits (see appendix).

New Findings Regarding the Medicines for Bipolar Illness

Physicians are becoming increasingly cautious when prescribing tricyclic antidepressants to persons with bipolar illness. Tricyclics are very effective medicines, especially for major depression, but there is some evidence that their use can increase the likelihood of "rapid cycling" (four or more episodes of mania or depression in a year). There is also concern that tricyclics can, at least temporarily, prevent a bipolar patient from experiencing the benefits of stabilization in those cases when lithium is used after the tricyclic. Since patients usually experience several bouts of depression before a manic episode and since patients often seek help when depressed and do not seek help when beginning a manic high, it was not uncommon in the past for the bipolar aspect of this depressive condition to go undetected for many years. Consequently, it was not unusual for lithium to be prescribed long after treatment by a tricyclic medication. More research is needed to discover if previous treatment with antidepressants interferes with the general efficacy of lithium in some persons with bipolar illness. Certainly, concomitant tricyclic antidepressants can interfere with lithium effectiveness if it is producing rapid cycling or mania.

The possible problems induced by tricyclics for people with bipolar illness is still one more reason why physicians are likely to prescribe one of the new SSRIs, such as Prozac. Since one-third of all people with serious depression have bipolar illness, cautious physicians realize that even though they may only see the patients in a down cycle, there may be an up cycle as well to their mood disorder.

MAO inhibitors are prescribed for patients during an acute episode of depression when the symptoms fit the category of atypical depression. They are usually used when other antidepressants have not worked. When they succeed where other medicines have not, it is like a miracle for the patient. Like all other antidepressants, MAO inhibitors can trigger mania in a patient with bipolar illness. It is unclear at this point whether MAO inhibitors are worse in that respect than others, but the problem does exist. Careful observation by health care professionals with insight from the family or friends of the client is very important.

Another current finding relates to dosage. A physician's monitoring of the level of lithium in a patient's blood has been focused in the past on maintaining a therapeutic level defined as .8 to 1.2. Dr. Modnes Schou's continued research into the efficacy of lithium reports that levels of .5 to .8 may actually be just as effective for most clients. Furthermore, levels as low as .3 can be helpful to elderly clients who do not metabolize medications as effectively as do younger patients.

Why is it so Important to Treat Persons with Bipolar Illness?

Physicians have reported that persons with bipolar illness experience some of the most painful depressions. These depressions are especially characterized by an inability to concentrate, a lack of ability to enjoy life, and thoughts of killing themselves.

Since bipolar patients usually have several bouts of depression before having an episode of mania, physicians often treat these clients for depression only. When the mania begins, many bipolar clients will self-medicate with alcohol (a depressant drug) as a means of calming themselves down. It is not surprising that 60 percent of bipolar patients are alcoholics. Since alcohol makes one less inhibited, it is a danger for anyone with frequent thoughts of suicide.

Mania is described as feeling high, and a time when the person eats and sleeps little. It sounds great, but the reality is that persons with bipolar illness suffer as much during their manic phases as they do when depressed. I learned about this not only from my experience with Ben, but unexpectedly from one experience of my own.

During the first years after Ben's death, I went through profound grief (a reactive depression). I had low energy, headaches, decreased ability to concentrate, intense sadness. Three years after his death, I volunteered to participate in a nationwide cancer prevention research project. Oncologists were attempting to discover if the drug tamoxifen would be effective in preventing breast cancer for women with specific risk factors. Soon after beginning the medication, I experienced an elevated mood and a decreased need to eat and sleep. One month after starting the medication, I reported these effects to the nurse working on the research project. Realizing that people often experience side effects when starting a medication and these effects often subside over time, I agreed to continue with the drug. However, I did warn her that if the side effects persisted for a long time or became more severe, I would stop the medication.

My elevated mood and decreased appetite appeared wonderful, especially to all of my friends who were envious of my weight loss and enjoyed my highly spirited conversation. What is hard to explain is the discomfort I was experiencing, especially during the nights when I got little sleep.

During the stages of grief following Ben's death, I often had difficulty sleeping. But the sleeplessness then was not as painful as it was during this manic episode. The only way I can begin to describe it is to say that I was excessively restless and just could not tolerate being in my body. I clearly remember the last night I was on the tamoxifen study. Perhaps I slept a total of one hour, but I cannot really be sure if I was able to sleep at all that night. I recall seeing the minutes slowly going by. I could not wait until 5 a.m. when I could get up and start working to take my mind off my discomfort.

Unlike people who suffer from manic episodes as part of their bipolar illness, I did not feel helpless about my situation. I knew that at 8 a.m. I could call the nurse to inform her I was discontinuing the medication. I realized that the effects of the medicine would gradually subside and I would again be able to sleep more normally. And unlike those who suffer from bipolar illness, my manic episode was not followed by the plunge into a painful depression.

Maintenance Medication for Frequent Recurring Unipolar Depression

Lithium is now found to be helpful to prevent or reduce the severity of future episodes of recurrent unipolar depression. There are two reasons why physicians consider its use. First, although antidepressants alone are very helpful during an acute bout of depression, they are discontinued after the depression subsides. If the depression is only a single episode or if the episodes are infrequent, the occasional use of an antidepressant may handle the problem. Unfortunately, for a substantial number of persons, episodes of unipolar depressions occur frequently. Lithium offers some protection against these future episodes.

Approximately one-third of persons with unipolar illness have frequently recurring episodes and will respond to lithium. Some researchers call these patients Unipolar II and believe them to have a form of bipolar illness. I personally believe that many people with Unipolar II are dysthymic most of the time. Their hypomanic cycles get them into what persons without depression experience as "feeling normal," and their depressive periods are very painful. Giving a stabilizing medication to Unipolar II patients reduces unnecessary suffering.

Second, taking lithium may decrease the likelihood of suicide for persons with unipolar depression, just as it has for those persons with bipolar illness, who become more stabilized with its use. One fact stands out in this regard. The two major classes of antidepressants (the tricyclic and MAO inhibitors) were developed in the mid 1950's. If antidepressants protected patients from suicide, one would expect the suicide rate to have declined as more depressed persons use these medicines. Unfortunately, the rate of suicide has not shown a substantial decline in the past decades, and the rate among young people has dramatically increased. Although the use of antidepressants has not increased the suicide rate, neither have they offered protection. Lithium is a medication that has decreased the likelihood that people with bipolar illness will kill themselves.

This issue is complex. Because suicide rates are affected by multiple factors (including cultural and methodologies used in assessing the rates) it has been difficult to determine if any medicine actually decreases the rates of suicide in persons with unipolar illness. Some research has shown antidepressants are equal to lithium for the maintenance treatment of unipolar depression. In the past there has also been some hesitancy to use lithium to prevent frequent recurrences of unipolar depression because there were fears it would adversely affect kidney function. Dr. Schou and others have carefully followed patients who have taken lithium for as many as twenty to thirty years and have not found a basis for concern. It is true that anyone who already has kidney disease may not be able to use lithium, but these patients cannot use salt either. There was one incident of a seventy-two year old male who developed kidney failure after being on lithium. This instance may be merely a coincidence since kidney disease is not uncommon and is on the rise worldwide. To be cautious, physicians monitor kidney function routinely for patients who take lithium.

TRICYCLIC ANTIDEPRESSANTS

The Story Behind the Discovery

The discovery of tricyclics did not initially involve psychiatry but developed in a roundabout way. Fieve writes that a French surgeon wanted to prevent surgical shock. He tried an antihistamine which did not have the results he wanted but did produce a calming effect on the patient. Other doctors wished to use medicines that would work like an antihistamine to help their surgical patients, so chemists began to create similar medicines. The result was chlorpromazine, a medication that is ultimately helpful in treating schizophrenia. Chemists often design medicines that are more effective and have fewer side effects by altering or adding to the chemical formulation of existing medicines. A Swiss chemist attempting to improve chlorpromazine produced Tofranil (imipramine). Tofranil is not effective for the treatment of schizophrenia, but it did relieve the symptoms of depression.

In short, a French surgeon's use of an antihistamine to prevent surgical shock prompted a Swiss chemist's attempt to improve on chlorpromazine, which produced the antidepressant imipramine. These lucky accidents show how many significant discoveries are made. Someone is looking for one thing and they come upon something else. Wasn't Christopher Columbus searching for the Indies when he stumbled on the Western Hemisphere? Improvements and advancement in science and medicine occur when open minded people discover something other than what they set out to find, and recognize the value of what they have stumbled upon.

The Use of Tricyclic Medications

One of the most practical ways to describe the different classes of antidepressants is to correlate them with the type of depressive symptoms they are most effective in treating. Tricyclic antidepressants are especially helpful to patients with major depression. The word "major" describes **typical** cases of serious depression. It defines patients who:

1. *experience low mood which is not relieved by any cheerful changes in the environment,*
2. *fall asleep without trouble, wake early and cannot get back to sleep,*
3. *feel worse in the morning,*
4. *have decreased appetite resulting in weight loss,*
5. *have difficulty concentrating,*
6. *have depressions that occur in discrete episodes.*

Tricyclic medications are helpful for major depression and have a success rate of at least 80 percent. There are many tricyclics on the market, and physicians may need to try several before discovering exactly which one will work best for a particular client. There is no way to know in advance or to test a patient to discover which tricyclic will prove to be most helpful. The oldest one and the one that has had the most rigorous investigation through the years is Tofranil (imipramine).

A tricyclic (as the word tricycle denotes) has a "three-ring chemical structure" (5/4/87, p. 52). Many physicians and their patients feel comfortable with the use of tricyclics, such as imipramine, because the medication has been around for almost forty years. The long-term effects of taking this medication have been studied. To date there is no evidence of problems resulting from continued use. Also, the extensive research on imipramine over the years has repeatedly proven its efficacy. Just a few years ago it was part of the large, multisite collaborative study by the National Institute of Mental Health. The results of the study indicated that a high percentage of patients who received medication combined with short term psychotherapies designed specifically for depression had successful outcomes.

MAO INHIBITORS

The Story Behind the Discovery

The story of the monoamine oxidase (MAO) inhibitors is a tale of still another lucky accident. This time it involved physicians in tuberculosis hospitals. They observed that the antibiotic created for tubercular patients had the effect of improving the mood of those who were depressed.

Monoamine oxidase (MAO) is an enzyme which causes the breakdown of many neurotransmitters once they get to the next neuron. MAO inhibitors prevent the breakdown of the neurotransmitters; thus, it increases the amount of neurotransmitters available in the brain. A tricyclic like imipramine also increases the amount of available neurotransmitters. It does this by preventing norepinephrine from being reabsorbed by presynaptic neurons.

So, in very simplistic terms, the tricyclics work by blocking reabsorption of the messengers by the nerve cells that release them, and the MAO inhibitors work to prevent the breakdown of neurotransmitters by the neurons that receive the message. It may appear as if scientists now "know" how these medicines work, but all that can be said is that although scientists do not fully understand how tricyclics and MAO inhibitors work to relieve depression, these medicines "bolster the actions of serotonin and norepinephrine, two of the chemicals that transmit impulses through the nervous system." (3/26/90, p. 39)

The Use of MAO Inhibitors

Again, the most practical way to begin talking about this class of anti-depressant drug is to describe the type of depression it helps. The term **atypical** depression does not describe a less serious or unusual kind of depression as compared to major depression. Instead, the term "atypical depression" describes patients who:

1. *can be temporarily cheered by a pleasant change in the environment,*

2. *are on an emotional rollercoaster in which praise and attention produce excessive highs and rejection or criticism produce extreme lows,*

3. *overeat and subsequently gain weight,*

4. *oversleep, and even after sleeping as much as twelve or fourteen hours will report feeling tired,*

5. *have decreased energy and lack motivation,*

6. *feel worse at the end of the day,*

7. *are less episodic and may report feeling constantly out of sorts.*

Two of the most commonly prescribed MAO inhibitors are Parnate and Nardil. Everyone experiences various side effects. Nardil usually causes more weight gain (a problem persons with atypical depression, like Ben, already struggle with). Parnate causes more disturbance in sleep patterns (a problem that is troublesome for many people with depression). It is paradoxical that even though MAO inhibitors have a success rate of at least 80 percent for clients with atypical depression, the medicine produces similar symptoms of the condition itself. Success rates for treatment of depression are impressively high, but my experience with Ben has made me aware of the need to be sympathetic and alert to the struggles of patients with the side effects of their treatment.

Selective Serotonin Reuptake Inhibitors

The Story Behind their Development

I know of no lucky accident involving Prozac (fluoxetine), one of the first SSRIs. With the large number of persons suffering from depression and the problems they encounter with side effects from tricyclics and MAO inhibitors, there was a need for medications that patients could and would take more easily. Even though the antidepressants discovered in the 1950's have an impressively high success rate, the efficacy of the tricyclics and MAO inhibitors are irrelevant if patients are unable or unwilling to stay on the medicine.

Tricyclics, for example can cause

1. *dry mouth*
2. *headache*
3. *sluggishness*
4. *dizziness*
5. *blurred vision*
6. *constipation*
7. *memory loss*
8. *insomnia*
9. *agitation*
10. *weight gain*

In addition, they can cause blood pressure and heart disturbances. This is especially a problem for older patients.

Often these side effects are mild and go away after a short period of time, but some people are unusually sensitive to them. Typically, about one-third of patients cannot or choose not to tolerate these side effects and discontinue the use of tricyclic medication.

The side effects of MAO inhibitors are much like the side effects from tricyclics. The big difference is that patients taking MAO inhibitors need to restrict their use of:

1. *some foods, e.g. aged cheese,*
2. *some medicines, e.g. cold medication,*
3. *some drinks, e.g. red wine.*

Because of the potentially harmful interactions of these products with an MAO inhibitor, physicians are careful to prescribe them only to clients who are able to follow the restrictions.

In additions to the side effects, tricyclics and MAO inhibitors require a patient to begin with a small dose and only gradually increase it. The therapeutic level is not reached for some time. Consequently, months may go by before the physician can accurately evaluate the suitability of a particular tricyclic or MAO inhibitor for a specific client. People who take Prozac, on the other hand, often get the maximum antidepressant effect from taking just the one 20 mg tablet which is given from the first day of treatment.

When Prozac became available in December of 1987 it soon became known as a wonder drug. It seemed like a wonder drug because it is easier to tolerate for most patients. Prozac, however, is not totally without side effects. The most common include:

1. *headaches*
2. *nausea*
3. *insomnia*
4. *jitteriness*
5. *weight loss*

It is that last side effect, weight loss, that may particularly explain the willingness of some patients to tolerate the other side effects of Prozac. Most of us are willing to lose a few pounds. In addition, we would rather feel slightly wired than sluggish. The side effects of Prozac are usually temporary, just as they are with other medications. Most people tolerate them well over the short period of time needed for the body to adjust to the medication.

Some Facts about SSRIs

1. SSRIs work like the tricyclics in that they block reabsorption of a neurotransmitter by the nerve cell that releases them. While tricyclics block reabsorption of a number of neurotransmitters, SSRIs work more exclusively on just one type of neurotransmitter -- serotonin. The term SSRIs refers to "selective serotonin reuptake inhibitors."

2. SSRI's help people with bipolar illness and those with atypical depression in a way that is similar to MAO inhibitors. Because there are no dietary restrictions with SSRIs, they are easier to use for these patients.

3. It is important to keep in mind that SSRIs are no more effective for depression than the tricyclics and MAO inhibitors. The older medications have a success rate of at least 80 percent. The success rate for the new SSRIs is not higher than the older medications.

4. Because SSRIs are easier to tolerate for most patients, they may be especially important for the elderly, whose bodies often have difficulty processing medication.

5. It is important to have normal levels of serotonin. Low serotonin levels are a predictor of suicidality because low levels of that particular neurotransmitter are associated with impulsivity and aggression.

Some Specifics about Prozac, Zoloft, Paxil, and Effexor

Prozac (fluoxetine) is a more wide range medication than some of the other SSRIs. Case reports indicate it may also be useful for patients suffering certain anxiety disorders, obsessive compulsive conditions, bulimia, kleptomania, obesity, addiction, and borderline personality disorder.

Zoloft (sertraline) works more on serotonin than Prozac but not as exclusively as does Paxil. Reseach indicated that it is helpful to patients with major depression.

Paxil (paroxetine) works exclusively on serotonin. Consequently, it is especially helpful for people whose depression manifests itself as symptoms of irritability and anger. There is also some indications that Paxil may be less likely to switch a person with bipolar illness from the depressive phase to mania.

Effexor (venlafaxine) is one of the newest SSRIs. Current hypotheses suggest that Effexor may work by two potential mechanisms of action, inhibiting the reuptake of both serotonin and norepinephrine.It may work as well for people suffering from severe typical depression as does the older tricylic, while producing fewer side affects than they do.

Because SSRIs are relatively new medicines, the long term affects are still not known. Physicians who choose to use them for extended periods will want to routinely reevaluate the long-term usefulness of these medicines for each of their clients.

Rationale for Caution

There is enthusiasm for the relatively low side effects of the SSRIs. There is no need to restrict the use of certain products when taking a SSRI as is required with the MAO Inhibitors. SSRIs users do not need to have their blood levels monitored as is done when taking lithium. SSRIs may seem like dream medications, but caution is warranted.

First, tricyclics and MAO inhibitors have been around for forty years and thus have a track record, which SSRIs do not. We cannot possibly know the long term consequences of using SSRIs . There does not appear to be any reason to suggest that use over long periods of time will prove to be problematic, especially since the other antidepressants have not. But until the data actually exists, no one can be certain.

Perhaps an even more interesting question is, will SSRIs continue to have an antidepressant effect for those clients who require on-going treatment? Or, will it become less effective with continued use? Until patients have been on a medication for many years, no one can say with certainty what the long term effect will be.

Third, no drug works perfectly for every one. Like any other medication, it is possible to have a paradoxical effect (patients getting worse rather than better). Furthermore, some SSRI users report feeling restless and some have tremors.

Most depression is treated by non-psychiatric physicians (e.g. internists, family practitioners, etc.). Since SSRIs are easier to prescribe, they tend to have greater success with it. But SSRIs, like any other medication, can produce adverse reactions.

Because depression is such a painful condition, compassionate doctors are willing to prescribe medications like Prozac, which has few side effects and helps most of those who take it. But unless they insist that patients produce some data on their moods, they may open themselves up to the same type of criticism with SSRIs as doctors experienced when valium and librium were prescribed widely for anxiety during the 1960's and 1970's.

Personal Comments Regarding Prozac

Prozac is a medication recommended for persons whose symptoms are that of atypical depression and who are not likely to follow the restrictions necessary for treatment with an MAO inhibitor. Ben's symptoms fit the diagnosis of atypical depression, and he was unlikely to stay away from pizza, lasagna, tacos and other foods prepared with cheese. Prozac was also ideal for Ben because it is recommended for patients with panic attacks, and it would not exacerbate Ben's weight problem. Prozac is also used for some clients who are phobic. Ben appears to have been an ideal candidate for treatment with Prozac.

My son died while taking Prozac. Do I blame his death on this medication? My answer today is "probably not," but six months after Ben's death, after hearing of reports of cases of persons using the medication becoming manic or suicidal, I did become concerned about the safety of this new medication.

Over time I have learned that Prozac, like any other antidepressant, must be prescribed differently for bipolar patients than for unipolar patients. There is a fundamental difference in the length of time a typical patient with unipolar depression will stay on the antidepressant, compared to the length of time a patient with bipolar illness usually needs to take that type of medicine. Persons with unipolar depression need to stay on their antidepressant for many months after their spirits rise. This is mandatory because depressive illness affects the body in many different ways. A change in mood is one of the first changes to be experienced after the medicine is started. But the depressive illness itself still affects people after their mood rises. Stopping the medicines before they are completely well increases the likelihood they will feel depressed again soon because their bodies are not yet fully recovered from the illness. It may be analogous to stopping an antibiotic prematurely because one begins to feel better. Antibiotics need to be taken for the full seven to ten days as prescribed by the doctor. Likewise, antidepressants need to be taken for several months (perhaps as many as nine months) after the patient's mood rises for persons who have unipolar depression.

Bipolar patients, on the other hand, typically will discontinue the use of one of these four classes of antidepressants a few weeks after their spirits rise. This is done in order to prevent them from being pushed into a manic episode. It is valuable for the physician to have as a working hypothesis the possibility that any depressed patient may turn out to actually have bipolar illness. This involves being conscientious about carefully following the mood cycles of anyone on an antidepressant. The best way to do this is to have the person, and sometimes the family or a close friend, keep a mood chart. This is simply done by scoring their mood each day from

+ 10 for extreme high,

0 for normal mood,

- 10 for deep low.

This easy system can detect moodswings and provide the kind of objective information that will save time, money, and unnecessary pain for everyone.

THE FOURTH CLASS - WELLBUTRIN

Wellbutrin (bupropion) became available in the summer of 1989. It is chemically unrelated to any other class of antidepressant. The 1993 Physicians Desk Reference states that "The neurochemical mechanism of the antidepressant effect of buproprion is not known." In a recent lecture, Dr. Frederick Goodwin stated that Wellbutrin likely acts on dopamine. It produces a stimulating effect on the central nervous system. It is helpful to a different group of people than those taking SSRIs.

Use for Students with ADHD

Young persons with attention deficit hyperactive disorder (ADHD) are typically helped by using Ritalin, a stimulant medication. ADHD is characterized by impulsivity, an inability to concentrate, and overactivity. Stimulant medication improves an ADHD student's ability to focus on a task while not exacerbating the hyperactivity. Ritalin does not cure ADHD, any more than insulin cures diabetes. It only allows the patient to manage a condition for which there is no cure.

Wellbutrin is being used as an alternative to Ritalin for students with ADHD. There is some enthusiasm for its use, but it is too soon to know if Wellbutrin will prove to be a more desirable medicine for ADHD than Ritalin. Since some children with ADHD are actually suffering from the manifestations of bipolar illness, Wellbutrin may prove to be a useful treatment. Wellbutrin has been found helpful for some children and adolescents who have both ADHD and depression symptoms, but may not be helpful for persons with high level anxiety.

Use of Wellbutrin for Adults

Wellbutrin is recommended for bipolar patients and for clients with major depression. Initial data indicate it may have less tendency to produce hypomania and mania than other antidepressants and therefore may be especially useful for patients with bipolar depression who often get manic when treated with antidepressants.

The side effects of Wellbutrin include:

1. *restlessness*
2. *agitation*
3. *insomnia*
4. *headache*
5. *nausea*
6. *vomiting*
7. *rash*

This list is not that different from what is found with the other antidepressants. Like the SSRIs, Wellbutrin does not cause weight gain. Initially, patients may even lose a few pounds.

The biggest concern is a risk of seizures. There have been some incidents in which the medication precipitated seizures. It is not a medication that should be prescribed for patients with a known diagnosis of epilepsy, or for those who have brain structural lesions, or those who have eating disorders, because people with these problems are at risk for seizures on Wellbutrin.

There are some indications that this stimulant medication may be especially helpful for elderly patients. Wellbutrin is sometimes prescribed to adults along with an SSRI because it may help to counteract the reduced sexual response that can occur with taking an SSRI.

A Personal Note on Wellbutrin

In the summer of 1989, Ben appeared to have been a perfect candidate for Wellbutrin. He had ADHD and was bipolar. However, it became available after Ben's death on May 31.

How would Ben have responded to Wellbutrin if he had had the opportunity to use it? I will never know the answer to that question. I do, however, know how his father responded to it when it was prescribed for his depression in 1990. You will recall that the response of a close relative (with a naturally high likelihood of having a similar body chemistry) is a good predictor of a patient's response to the same medicine. Garry's response to Wellbutrin was not successful. This has taught me that no matter how ideal candidates may originally seem to be for a particular medicine, there is no guarantee that it will work for them. In 1994 I now know why Ben probably would not have responded well to Wellbutrin. Ben had a serious anxiety disorder.

NEW VERSUS OLD MEDICATION

Advertising and commercials have conditioned us to equate the newness of a product with improvement. It has gotten to the point that established products almost have to claim they are in some way new and improved if they are to continue to hold their customers. The term "tried and true" does not hold the same meaning in our era of rapid change as it did when change was less dramatic and ongoing.

The older anti-depressants have been around for nearly forty years. The tricyclics are still very effective medications for some people with severe cases of major depression. MAO inhibitors are still effective for some persons with depression when all other medicines have failed.

Lithium was used 1800 years ago to treat or promote the physical and mental well being of patients. Working on the second messenger system, it is the only medication that can function as an amplifier when the person is depressed and as a minimizer when the person become hypomanic or manic. Lithium also augments the effectiveness of other antidepressants. Some psychiatrists are so convinced of the augmentative value of lithium that they will routinely give it to all their unipolar patients along with the antidepressant, and then remove it once the antidepressant has relieved the symptoms.

The new SSRI's will most likely prove to be a great blessing for millions. It has been said that only one out of four persons with severe depressive illness sought treatment for their illness. In recent years, the figure comes closer to one out of two. In part this is a result of efforts by organizations like the National Institute of Mental Health, which has worked to raise the public awareness of the symptoms of depression. Undoubtedly it is also due in part to the development of the new, easier to tolerate, SSRIs.

Each year pharmaceutical companies produce more new medications that have proven, in controlled trials, to be efficatious. Put on the market for use by the general public, they may prove over time to be effective for a large number of people. Examples of these are:

Remeron (mirtazapine) Functions like the SSRI's, but does not cause the sexual dysfunction that a minority of patients experience as a side effect. Its pharmacologic action includes improving activity of norepinephrine and serotonin.

Risperdal (resperedone) Originally developed as a front-line medication treatment option for psychotic disorders, but is proving to be helpful in producing stability for some bipolar patients who do not respond to lithium.

Zyprexa (olanzapine) A new front-line medication for treatment of psychotic disorder, it produces fewer side effects than older anti-psychotic medication. It may prove to be helpful to schizo-affective patients. It does not have the side affect of reducing bone marrow.

Revia (naltrexone) Purported to work for people who are both alcoholic and depression, it works on the brain morphine systems. It may be helpful for adolescent-onset alcoholism.

Luvox (fluvoxamine maleate) An SSRI of a new series, it is chemically unrelated to the other SSRI's. It is especially helpful for people who suffer from obsessive compulsive disorder.

Neurontin (gabapentin) Early research indicates two-thirds of bipolar I and II patients sustained mood-stabilizing effects. It has a good side affect profile.

Lamitcal (lamotrigine) May have antidepressant properties in bipolar I and II depression, in patients resistant to standard mood stabilizers and antidepressants.

When starting an antidepressant, patients will need to know what to expect. It is likely that they will experience a jagged rather than straight-line improvement in their symptoms. They may feel better, then worse, better, then worse. But their course will be upwards over time, if the medicine is effective for them. Only a trial of medication will actually tell what works most effectively for a specific person. Careful follow-up with a physician is essential.

One thing is clear. Mental illness, left untreated, costs twice as much in real dollars as treatment. All other illnesses cost the same whether you treat them or not. Isn't the treatment of mental illness the most cost effective medicine there is?

Suicide

Suicide is not a rare occurrence or a minor health concern. "Approximately 30,000 people of all ages kill themselves annually in the United States." ("Useful," 1986) This translates into 73 people each day. Suicide can occur when people perceive themselves as having an irresolvable life crisis.

The issue of loss is often involved. It may be the loss of one's health, the loss of loved ones, the loss of the financial means to continue a certain life style, or any other important loss. Losses are common for persons as they get older. Having a chronic, perhaps ultimately fatal illness like cancer is more likely as you get older. Your chances of seeing your close relatives and lifelong companions die is more likely in later years. People on fixed incomes may struggle to retain previous lifestyles. Historically, suicide has been highest among the elderly and lowest among the young.

SUICIDE IN THE YOUNG

Today the situation is changing. "Suicide for the elderly has somewhat declined, while the rate has soared for adolescents and young adults." ("Useful," 1986) "For adolescents, in 1950, the rate of suicide per 100,000 population was 2.7; by 1980, it had reached 8.5. This constitutes an increase of 215 percent. Suicide rates in this group appear to have increased again in the mid-1980's; by 1985, the rate per 100,000 was 10.0." (Hoberman, 1989) Furthermore, although older adolescents and young adults are more at risk for suicide than are younger adolescents and children, most recently, the suicide rate for these younger persons has risen sharply. One study indicates the "suicide rate among 10 - 14 year olds increased relatively little between 1960 and 1981; however, between 1980 and 1985, the rate for this group doubled." (Hoberman, 1989).

It always takes some time to compile the data on any condition. The Fall, 1993 issue of the Lifesavers Newsletter gave the most recent statistics on the suicide rate for the young. Dr. David Shaffer reports,"In 1991, 1,899 teenagers committed suicide and the rates (18/100,000 for boys and 3.7/100,000 for girls) are substantially the same as in 1988, when the rate for youth suicide reached an all time peak." The data also indicates that during the past 15 years, the rate of suicide for girls has remained relatively the same, whereas, the rate for boys has tripled.

The age of onset of depression has declined. Before World War II, the age of onset of a severe depressive episode typically occurred somewhere in middle age, late forties or early fifties. Since World War II, the first onset of a major depressive episode usually occurs somewhere in the late 20's or early 30's. (Gelman, 1987, p. 48).

Bipolar disturbance represents an estimated one-third of those suffering from serious depression. Bipolar illness has an early onset. The average age of onset for a first psychiatric episode for many kids with this and other forms of serious depression is 10 to 11 years old. (Hoberman, 1989, p. 9). My son was diagnosed at the Mayo Clinic as suffering from depression. Before going to Mayo he saw a local psychiatrist because I felt he clearly showed symptoms of depression. Both of these appointments occurred when Ben was eleven years old.

The possibility of suicide in a young person is frightening to all parents. Unpredictable and seemingly incomprehensible, it makes everyone feel vulnerable. I do not know how often I have heard people tell parents of a suicide victim how much they fear something like this happening in their own family. We live with the fact that 18 adolescents kill themselves in the United States every day. Suicide is the second leading cause of death for people between the ages of 15 and 24 years. (Larson, 1990, p. 1019)

CHILDREN AT RISK

In an interview for "Lifesaver Newsletter," (1993) psychiatrist Dr. Cynthia Pfeffer reports that "118 U.S. children 5 to 14 years old committed suicide in 1968, producing the very low rate of 0.3 per 100,000...By 1989, the childhood suicide rate more than doubled, and suicide advanced to the sixth leading cause of death for children in this age group." Parents and teachers want to know which children are especially at risk. Pfeffers says,

> Male children - like male adults - commit suicide more frequently than do females, and those with serious psychiatric illnesses, impaired relationships, limited adaptive skills, and extensive social problems are particularly vulnerable to future suicidal behavior. The psychiatric symptoms that especially flag suicidal children are indicators of depression: sadness, irritability, aggressive behavior, preoccupation with death, poor concentration, and withdrawal from friends and schools. Children with serious mood disorders remain at high risk later in life, and studies find that they have high rates of suicide attempts as adolescents and high rates of suicide as young adults.

ADOLESCENTS AT RISK

Dr. Garfinkel's book, <u>Adolescent Suicide</u>, gives a comprehensive overview of current research identifying the young people who are especially at risk of completing suicide. He cites the 1988 work by Brent, et al. who describe the psychiatric disorders of young people who completed suicide.

They found that 93 percent of the victims in the study had at least one major psychiatric diagnosis. Various types of depressive illnesses were the most common type of psychiatric disorder at the time of death. Forty one percent were diagnosed as having a severe depression disorder, 22 percent were rated as having dysthymia (mild but continuous low mood) and 7 percent were seen as experiencing a manic or hypomanic episode. Other common diagnoses at the time of death were as follows: substance abuse (41 percent); attention deficit disorder (26 percent); conduct disorder (22 percent); and anxiety disorder (15 percent) (Hoberman, 1989).

As important as these finding are, another factor emerged: co-morbidity. The existence of two or more conditions especially increases risk. Young people with serious depression *and* an anxiety disorder, particularly if they suffer from panic attacks, produce a combination that puts them at great risk. Adolescents and young adults with a serious anxiety disorder *and* alcohol/drug use are at high risk. Young schizophrenics who *also* experience the onset of a depressive episode have an elevated risk for suicide.

My son had a complex and serious depressive disorder, an anxiety disorder which included panic attacks and an attention deficit disorder. Co-morbidity is especially seen in people with bipolar illness, but not exclusively. His bipolar illness co-morbid with anxiety disorder and ADD makes him an appropriate example of a typical young person at elevated risk for completing suicide. Was substance abuse an issue for him? His single but unusual drinking incident makes me wonder if he did not have the potential for developing a problem in this area. If he had, he would have been like so many others who use it to self-medicate the anxiety so frequently associated with depression.

ATTEMPTERS VS COMPLETERS

Historically, there are two factors distinguishing people who attempt suicide as compared to those who complete suicide. First is the type of condition they suffered. Attempters were described as having neurosis or personality disorders rather than combinations of depression, anxiety, substance abuse, or schizophrenia.

The other factor found between attempters and completers is a gender difference. Females attempt suicide four times as often as do males ("Useful," 1986), but more men are likely to complete suicide than are females. "Males account for three-fourths of all committed suicide." ("Useful," 1986). Youthful suicide is particularly dominated by males; the rate is nearly five times that of females. Furthermore, the rate of suicide between 1950 and 1980 has increased 295 percent for males, whereas the rate for females has only increased by 67 percent (Hoberman, 1989).

In recent years, a third factor has emerged -- the availability of a lethal weapon. The presence of a gun in the home elevates risk, especially for adolescents and young adults. Brent and Perper note that from 1933 (the Great Depression) to 1982 the rate of suicide in the United States for 10 - 24 year olds increased 1.3 fold while the rate in firearms suicide for that group rose 2.4 fold. They further report that suicide rates are lower in those parts of the country where fewer people own guns.

It is important to remember that typically 15 percent of people suffering from serious co-morbid conditions (depression, anxiety, drug/alcohol abuse and schizophrenia) will use whatever means is available to end their lives. However, the presence of an easily available firearm may, on the other hand, increase the risk that an uninhibited, impulsive young person without a serious psychiatric disorder will act on a sudden suicidal impulse.

When thinking about the difference between attempters and completers, it is a mistake to think a person who has a history of attempts will never complete it. Information from the Department of Health tells us: "People who have made serious suicide attempts are at highest risk for actually killing themselves. The suicide rate for repeat attempters is up to 643 times higher than the overall rate in the general population. Between 20 - 50 percent of the people who commit suicide had previously made attempts." ("Useful," 1986)

The increase in suicide among young people may be resulting from the combination of earlier onset of depressive illness, the increased rate of depression at this particular time in history, and an increase in ownership of guns.

WHAT ARE YOUNG ATTEMPTERS OR COMPLETERS TRYING TO DO?

You might think the answer to the question is obvious. The suicidal person wants to die. But this may not be true for many adolescents. "In a recent study of Minnesota teenagers, 64 percent of suicide attempters said they really did not want to die".

("Supporting," 1986). In fact, "Follow-up studies (of persons who attempted but did not complete suicide) reveal their intense ambivalence about dying. Not only are they glad to be alive, but for many, a suicide attempt marked a turning point. It was a dramatic signal that their problems demanded serious and immediate attention. Most of those who survived their suicide attempts indicated that what they really wanted was a change in their lives ("Useful," 1986).

That to me is the key; they wanted a change in their lives. Joseph Campbell (1990) gives us some insight into this. He says,

> The New Testament teaches dying to one's self, literally suffering the pain of death to the world and its values. This is the vocabulary of the mystics. Now, suicide is also a symbolic act. It casts off the psychological posture that you happen to be in at the time, so that you may come into a better one. You die to your current life in order to come to another of some kind. But, as Jung says, you'd better not get caught in a symbolic situation. You don't have to die, really, physically. All you have to do is die spiritually and be reborn to a larger way of living.

You do not have to literally die to change your life. When I say that what my son did was stupid, I mean Ben took an idea that is symbolically true and acted it out literally. Or as the famous psychiatrist Carl Jung might have said, the best way to die to one way of life and to be born to a new, larger way of life is to change your attitude.

Committing suicide is an especially powerful idea in the mind of many adolescents. Evidence for this is found in the statistics on suicide attempters. When the data from all age groups are compared, there are approximately ten attempts for every one completed suicide. But when you look at attempts versus completions for young people, "the ratio for youth is 25 - 50 suicide attempts for every one suicide completion" ("Useful, " 1986).

Suicide is a symbolic act which speaks to the psychological issue for young people in their particular stage of life. Adolescence is a time of putting aside one way of life, i.e., childhood, and being re-born into a new way of life, i.e., adulthood. The theme of transition is a strong force in the adolescents' minds and it is easy to see how they may physically act out their psychological process. It is lucky for all of us that there are 25 - 50 attempts for every completed suicide. These young people have a chance to see that the goal was change rather than death.

PREVENTION PROGRAMS OF THE PAST

"Several studies have demonstrated that suicide prevention programs have not made a significant impact on the rate of suicides." In recent years, a number of suicide prevention curricula have been developed specifically targeted to youth. Dr.Garfinkel notes the curricula of these programs tend to focus on the circumstances surrounding suicides (Hoberman, 1989, pp. 22-23). This is not effective because "suicide victims kill themselves when confronted with typical stress situations that most of us face without major difficulty. Stressors alone do not likely pose a risk for the adolescent. Instead, it appears to be the existence of stressors for particular individuals with pre-existing psychiatric conditions that create a climate of risk."

In my son's case, the stressor may have been his pile of unfinished school work. He was given exactly the same assignments everyone else got. The difficulty arose from his own inability to finish the work the rest of the class managed to complete on time. Procrastination is a common characteristic of persons with depressive illness. This, plus the cognitive difficulties associated with his depression, ADHD, and anxiety all contributed to create the pile of unfinished work.

Rather than being a logical act growing out of an impossible life situation, adolescent suicide is often an impulsive act. Garfinkel puts it this way: "The seemingly impulsive, crisis-nature of the actual suicide is impressive. Relatively few suicides showed evidence of advance planning or even precautions against being stopped or discovered at the time of the act." (Hoberman, 1989, p. 17)

WARNING SIGNS

Suicide prevention in the past has often focused on looking for warning signs. These signs include:

(1) Previous Suicide attempts
People who have made serious suicide attempts are at high risk for actually killing themselves.

(2) Suicide talk
People who commit suicide often talk about it first. Statements like, "They'd be better off without me," or "No one will have to worry about me much longer," can be give-aways. A more offhand "I've had it," may also be a clue.

(3) Making arrangements
Some suicidal individuals take steps to put their affairs in order. They draw up or alter their wills, give away prized possessions, make arrangements for pets, or otherwise act as if they are preparing for a trip. They talk vaguely about going away.

(4) Personality or Behavior Change
A normally buoyant person may seem increasingly down for no apparent reason. There may be a loss of interest in school, work, friends, hobbies, and recreational activities that gave them pleasure in the past. They may begin to express a sense of worthlessness or hopelessness, or excessive guilt.

(5) Clinical Depression
While 85 percent of depressed people are not suicidal, most of the suicide-prone are depressed. ("Useful," 1986, pp. 15-16)

The Use of Warning Signs

The question is: Although these signs are frequently present before a suicide, are they easily detected by others in the environment? To answer this, I think about my son's death. Any previous attempts Ben may have made were not done in a manner that I recognized as warnings. He did tell his therapist early in treatment that he had pointed a gun at his head. When she told me this, it was news to me. He probably fooled around dangerously with guns but never did this when adults were around. Ben's accident-prone behavior throughout his life seems now to be an ongoing flirtation with danger.

His suicide talk consisted of the remark, "A lot you'd care if something happened to me." This statement was made in the context of our conversation about his over-eating. I did not catch it as suicidal talk. Did he put affairs in order? He had cleaned his room the week before, but in preparation for a guest. We saw behavioral change, but this was expected with the change in medication he was undergoing. We thought his clinical depression had lifted and hoped his therapy could be reduced. He had been looking forward to things such as going to horse shows with his riding instructor and using the new saddle we just bought for his daily horseback riding.

When a surviving family member looks back on the last days of the life of a person who commits suicide, it is possible to pick up some clues. But at the time they are happening, these behaviors are not blatantly different from what is happening in the person's life on any other day. Someone once said that if President Kennedy had not been shot, no one would remember he was in Dallas in November of 1963. Likewise, if my son had not died I would not be able to recall what happened the last week in May, 1989.

Dr. Garfinkel cautions against an over-emphasis on precipitating events, the presence of stressors, or signs of plans to die. The impulsive nature of suicide in young people makes preventing particular suicides unlikely (Hoberman, 1989). What I have learned in the last few years leads me to agree with that assertion. People I have met in suicide survivors' support groups indicate there were few, if any, distinct indications their loved ones were contemplating suicide. These people are loving, bright individuals. Most of them, like myself, did not have a clue their loved one was at risk of committing suicide. The victim did not *clearly* display many of the warning signs of suicide, nor did their behavior seem dramatically different on the day it occurred or in the weeks preceding the death.

Asking adults to be alert to signs and making them responsible for prevention places an unrealistic and consequently unfair burden on them. Research indicates "There is no profile or checklist for identifying a suicidal person. Suicide, like much of human behavior, is difficult to predict. Despite their best efforts, even experts cannot say whether or when a person will try to commit suicide" ("Useful," 1986).

An over-emphasis on the stressors immediately preceding a person's death not only prevents us from having a clear understanding of the cause of the problem, which is the psychiatric illness, but when we overemphasize the preceding stressor it may cause the survivors to torture themselves unnecessarily.

After a suicide, survivors often say, "If only I had done this or if I had done that the suicide may have been prevented." The person's suicide may have had little to do with the individual's outer life situation. Recent work comparing the lives of those who kill themselves, those who attempted, and those who died of natural causes reveals that, in the main, the lives of those who kill themselves are often no worse than those of others who carry on. To the objective outsider, their situations are far from hopeless, and there are ways other than suicide to solve their problems. ("Useful," 1986) It is not so much the circumstances of a person's life, but the pain of their illness which is relevant.

Rather than trying to prevent suicide by looking for warning signs or focusing on the preceding stressor or trigger, it seems more logical to focus on the cause, namely the psychiatric conditions. Emphasizing the diagnosis and treatment of depression, anxiety disorder, and drug/alcohol abuse makes sense. These are very common and treatable disorders.

It may seem paradoxical for me to advocate the importance of diagnosis and treatment of these conditions since my own child completed suicide while seeing a therapist on a regular basis. Research does, however, indicate treatment as a factor helpful in reducing risk. We sought the best treatment program available in our region. I feel strongly that Ben's therapist is one of the finest adolescent psychiatrists in our state. She had excellent rapport with him. Ben always reported feeling so much better after seeing her, and we felt there were many results from each of their sessions. We were extremely lucky to have found an adolescent psychiatrist as knowledgeable as she was in the current research in mood disorder, and one who specialized in working with children and adolescents with this condition. Garry and I did not mind driving three hours to her office in another city and three hours back home again to get this level of care for our son. I do not blame my son's death on his therapist for not predicting when he would be suicidal. Suicide is an impulsive act. How is anyone going to predict when an impulsive act is going to occur?

Getting medical treatment for any illness does not necessarily mean the doctor is going to be able to "fix" the condition. If my son had cancer, no one would assume that getting medical treatment for his condition would guarantee survival. Bipolar illness, like cancer, is a very serious condition. For everyone who has the illness, it is a condition which requires a significant amount of care and monitoring. Historically, for approximately

20 percent of people with bipolar illness, the condition is fatal. Depression may be the common cold of psychiatry, but the difference between depression and a cold is that depression can kill you.

Depression in young persons has generally been undiagnosed and untreated. Although I recognize suicide has been with us throughout history and probably always will be, a more realistic goal is to increase the percentage of persons with depression receiving proper treatment for the condition. Although the number of adults seeking treatment for depression has improved in recent years, children and adolescents do not yet have the same level of care as is currently received by adults. Too many young people with mild to severe depression are suffering unnecessarily.

THE NEED FOR SCREENING

Teachers and health care professionals want to help prevent suicide in the young when possible. Unfortunately, studies indicate that teachers are in the same situation as parents. They also cannot easily detect the presence of depression in children or adolescents. Physicians likewise often do not identify depression in patients who complete suicide. "One study found that half to three-quarters of nonpsychiatrist medical doctors miss it." (Gelman, 1987) This finding indicates a need for the use of a screening device. Before outlining the use of screening, the following comments are important.

Although teachers can be helpful in identifying depression in children and adolescents, it may be unwise to mandate that they be held accountable for doing this. Past experience with government bureaucracy in enforcing accountability is as follows: If teachers are held responsible for identifying depression in their students

1. *some sort of rules and regulations will be promulgated*

2. *more paper work will be added to the work load of these already overburdened people, and*

3. *when a student, impulsively and without clear signs of distress, does commit suicide there may be efforts to produce blame.*

I think the last thing anyone wants to do is increase blame and guilt adults may feel when a youngster dies. Teachers are not trained to spot depressive illness, and it seems unfair to make them responsible.

I would like to suggest that this challenging health issue be handled like any other health problem: by a combination of professional persons and trained volunteers. I would like to draw a comparison between a screening that could be done for depression in junior and senior high and the routine vision and hearing screening done in elementary school.

What I am suggesting is something a few school systems are already doing. They give a simple paper and pencil test to their junior high and high school students. It would consist of having the pupils rate themselves (1-Most of the time 2-Sometimes, 3-never) on statements such as these:

1. *I sleep very well.*
2. *I feel like crying.*

3. *I get stomach aches.*
4. *I think life isn't worth living.*
5. *I am good at things I do.*
6. *I am easily cheered up.*
7. *I have lots of energy.*
8. *I feel very lonely.*
9. *I feel very bored.*
10. *I have horrible dreams*

Or, students could use an instrument similar to the Beck Depression Inventory. They would simply choose which phrase best describes how they feel. Here are example of two items on that questionnaire.

---

0 I get as much satisfaction out of things as I used to.
1 I don't enjoy things the way I used to.
2 I don't get real satisfaction out of anything anymore.
3 I am dissatisfied or bored with everything

0 I don't feel I am worse than anybody else.
1 I am critical of myself for my weaknesses or mistakes.
2 I blame myself all the time for my faults.
3 I blame myself for everything bad that happens.

Depression scales for adults have been used for some time. Self report scales on depression are generally found to be valid, can easily be done in a group setting, and take far less time than the individual vision and hearing screening currently done in our schools.

In making the comparison between sensory screening and depression screening, I hope that I will not be misunderstood. I commend the wonderful volunteers who unselfishly give of their time to do the important work of vision and hearing screening each year. But I would like to continue with this comparison between sensory screening and a possible screening for depression to make the point that, in my opinion, screening for depression has a greater priority. I hope you will forgive me if, as a bereaved parent, I state the case fairly strongly.

"In 1980 3,442 persons aged 15 - 19 committed suicide" (Hoberman, 1989). Did three or four thousand school aged youngster die in 1980 because they were slightly near-sighted or far-sighted? I am not aware of an alarming increased rate of hearing problems in this country. In contrast, the age of onset of depression seems to be occurring younger now than in years past. remember that in 1986, 39 percent of adolescents reported suffering from some level of depression. There is also a dramatic increase in the suicide rate for adolescents.

Hearing and vision screening is done because these problems could interfere with learning. Does not the "diminished ability to think or concentrate," "slowed thinking or indecisiveness," "loss of interest or pleasure in usual activities," "fatigue or loss of energy," "change in sleeping patterns," and the "feelings of worthlessness" that are associated with depression and which translate into the "decline in the quality of school work" also interfere with learning? Does not depressive illness interfere with learning just as much as problems with vision or hearing?

"Each year in the United States, approximately 5,000 young people age 24 and younger commit suicide ("Teen," 1985). We are not dealing with rare phenomena but with a significant public health problem which research indicates is generally undertreated.

The National Institute of Mental Health reports that undiagnosed and untreated, "Youngsters with this problem are left to their own resources in dealing with their illness. These young people often rely on passive or negative behaviors in their attempts to deal with problems" ("Adolescent," 1986). My son did not have a behavior problem in school, but he, like many other depressed kids, was passive. How many depressed youth develop behavior problems and are treated as "bad" rather than youngsters with an undiagnosed illness?

When the results of screening indicate the presence of depression, the students can be treated like anyone else with a medical problem. It is not the parents' fault when a youngster needs glasses to correct his vision. Why would we assume it is the parents' fault when a youngster needs treatment for depression?

A NO-BLAME APPROACH

General education about depression as a biological condition can be helpful, and it would decrease the blame associated with the condition. Many other illnesses used to have shame associated with them. Years ago, cancer was seen as something of which to be ashamed. In the past, attempts were made to hide the fact that a person had the disease; sometimes it was covered up as the cause of death on the death certificate. Today there is not any stigma of blame associated with cancer. We only think of persons with cancer as innocent victims of a cruel disease.

I feel it would be a positive step forward if the same could be done for depressive illness. I think all too often when family members hear that their loved one is depressed, it translates in their mind as: "What have I done to cause the problem?" Frequently, the environment had little to do with the illness.

Sitting in my suicide support group has been a real eye-opening experience for me. I look at the wonderful people sitting in that room with me, and it becomes perfectly clear these people have nothing to feel guilty about. This has helped me to put a measure of reality into my own situation. I could choose to be hard on myself and find ways to feel guilty about Ben's death. I would, however, never be that unobjective about other people. Seeing the contrast between how I could choose to think about my own situation and how I actually see other people, I have come to see that I too have no logical reason to feel guilty about his depression or his death.

It would be wonderful if other people when hearing the words, "your loved one may have a problem with depression" would not feel that it is somehow their fault. I think the most helpful way to do this is to stress the biochemical theories of depression. Getting scientific information helps us becoming objective.

IS REDUCTION OF THE SUICIDE RATE AN ATTAINABLE GOAL?

I do not know if we can reduce the number of suicides. I do not think it is wise to make it a goal. Not all suicides are preventable. Suicide is too complicated an issue to have one simple answer. A historical and worldwide perspective on suicide is useful.

Suicide is as old as it is universal. People have been killing themselves since the beginning of recorded time. Suicide has meant different things among various cultures through the ages. It has not always evoked horror. It is mentioned matter-of-factly in the Bible. It was tolerated, even honored, as a particularly decent death in ancient Greece and Rome. Suicide continues to be so honored in Asian and Middle Eastern societies today. It was the means to heaven for early Christian martyrs and is now believed by Islamic martyrs to be their ticket to salvation. Suicide has meant delivery from military defeat and escape from enslavement.

Suicide survived religious and secular transformation in the sixth century, as a sin against God and a crime against the community, to become a major theme for Renaissance writers. It was a cause for enlightenment philosophers and a fashion among melancholy nineteenth century romantics. In the last century, suicide captured the interest of mental health scientists, and the modern study of suicide got under way. What has been defended as an intellectual choice by enlightenment thinkers came to be seen as, if not a sign of mental illness, a means of relief from psychic pain and sorrow ("Useful," 1986).

Because it is unlikely that we have yet come to the final chapter in our discoveries about suicide, perhaps it is unwise to make any statement about the ability to reduce suicide. What is clear, however, is that we now have effective means of treating depression and that we have a large number of people who are not receiving it. Of the estimated 25 - 35 million people with severe depression, at least fifty percent are not getting treatment. Since at least 80 percent of severely depressed persons and probably nearly all of those with mild cases could be significantly helped with presently available methods of treatment, an aggressive approach to identification and treatment of depression seems to be a realistic goal. Maybe if we focused on that, the suicide rate would take care of itself. Even if it was not reduced, we as a nation may feel we did our best to deal with one of suicide's major causes. We would have helped to decrease the unnecessary suffering in our young people, the one group that has not had an increase in health care in the last 30 years.

To hear the phrase "suicide is preventable" is analogous to hearing that "cancer is curable." It may be more precise to say: Some types of cancer may be cured if detected early, if patients receive competent medical treatment, and if they are determined to survive. A sense of hope for the future is an important ingredient. Similarly, some people with depressive illness, anxiety disorder, schizophrenia, and those with some major traumatic loss or serious physical illness may be deterred from completing suicide if detected early and the patients receive competent medical treatment and finds within themselves an attitude of determination to survive. A sense of hope for the future is an important ingredient for them as well.

When thinking about death, we come back to a paradox. What my son did was an impulsive act, and his therapist quite correctly called it stupid. My son is not to be admired for his act, but for some mysterious reason I can not help but believe it was his fate. I always come back to the message I received as I stood over Ben's body: "This was supposed to happen this day."

WHEN EVERYTHING YOU'VE TRIED FEELS LIKE FAILURE

This book outlined an elective class designed to work with young people with depression and anxiety. Research indicates it has a good chance of working. This class should give hope to the many parents who struggle with children with emotional difficulties. By combining current advances in medicine with effective teaching, there is hope we can help the many young people who need it.

The success of the program for any given student will depend on how serious their emotional problems are and how multifaceted they are. Ben had three serious disorders. Helping him to cope with that combination of problems was extremely difficult. Helping any young person learn to cope with challenges is always difficult. Luckily, most cases of depression are unipolar and are not associated with a learning disability.

During my years as a college instructor, I taught a class entitled "The Psychology of the Exceptional Child." Each year I required the class to compare the various ways of working with exceptionally capable students. My students were also required to compare the techniques used to work with children who have problems with school. What they discovered is that almost anything done with capable youngsters works fairly well. Having gifted students skip a grade, or placing gifted students in special classrooms, or keeping them in their regular grade but giving them enrichment assignments can be successful for gifted students. Occasionally, even doing little if anything for them still works, because exceptionally capable youngsters often find ways of making good use of their time on their own. They will read or engage themselves in a hobby that teaches them useful things. Although no generalization is true for every child, most of the time whatever is done for gifted students is successful.

When my students analyzed strategies for working with children who have learning problems, they found a different picture. Putting these students in separate classrooms isolates them, preventing them from benefiting from the interaction they would get from capable classmates who can serve as role models. In an isolated situation, teachers may begin to expect less from them, and they in turn may begin to expect less of themselves. But if they are left in a classroom with no special help, they find it difficult to handle. If their learning problems are not understood, they do not feel comfortable. Repeating a grade usually does not benefit a child with learning problems.

Almost any method used with especially capable students has a good chance of working; whereas, no method of working with students with difficulties will necessarily guarantee success. We need to recognize that working with difficult kids is just plain hard work. And, no matter how hard we try to help these students, we may not succeed.

The methods we use need to match the problems they have. When I look back on Ben's life, I see how many of the things I did for Ben did not match his problem. Often I would advise him to concentrate harder. Continually asking a child with an attention deficit to concentrate is ridiculous. The inability to concentrate is the major characteristic of the condition. I also frequently told him to think about the consequences of his behavior before he acted. Impulsively is the second major characteristic of attention deficit. ADHD is a deficit of thinking, i.e., inability to concentrate and a lack of ability to plan.

On the other hand, some of the things I did to help Ben were exactly the right thing to do to meet his needs. Even this had limited success because of the seriousness of his condition. This book's many suggestions to help the parents and teachers of students with difficulties should not inadvertently become a weapon used to blame anyone when things do not work out well for the young person. When a student commits suicide, often the parents will say, "If only I had done this or that, things might have been different; we might have prevented the death." Even when things are done to help a student, it does not necessary follow that all of their problems will be solved.

It is important to have a balanced perspective on the techniques used to help young people with problems. It is not logical (or fair) to blame the youngster when things do not work out as we hoped. It is equally unfair to blame ourselves -- the parents, the teacher, the doctors who tried their best to help them. When I was crying after Ben's death and asking myself, "Wasn't there any way we could have saved him?", I concluded that if Ben's problems would have been easy, we probably would have been able to help him find a way. This also gave me a glimpse into Ben's thinking. He had been through many strategies and perhaps he concluded that nothing would ever work out for him.

The good news for most parents is that the vast majority of young people with emotional problems do not have a condition as complex or serious as Ben's. An analogy to vision problems is useful here. Some people are blessed with perfect vision, but it is very common for people to have a mild problem. A pair of glasses or contact lenses are usually enough to give the needed correction. Similarly, while most people never experience depression or anxiety disorder, perhaps as many as 40 percent of the adolescent population do have at least a mild form of depression often with concurrent anxiety. Some experience anxiety alone. At least 80 percent would be significantly helped by the cognitive and social skills training for their depression. Anxiety is treated with various coping strategies. Research tells us that these methods, with the use of medication when appropriate, can provide help to young people who need it.

For young people who are blind, glasses are ineffective. It is unfair to blame students with very serious vision impairments because they cannot see and because they do not respond favorably to a pair of glasses. Neither is it logical to say that glasses, in general, do not work simply because they are incapable of making the blind see. It is neither the doctor's fault nor the eye glass company's fault for failing to cure the blindness.

Similarly, there is a percentage of young people with severe or complex depressions. It is not their fault they do not respond favorably to the treatment programs that succeed in helping the majority who suffer from depression. Neither is it logical to say that cognitive and social skills training for depression and techniques to cope with anxiety are not effective because some youngsters still take their own lives even after participating in these kinds of programs. It is unfair to blame psychiatrists who undoubtedly suffer enormously when some of their patients choose suicide.

Paradoxically, although medication relieves the symptoms of depression for most people who take them, it is not clear that they curb the rate of suicide. Antidepressants were first developed in the mid 1950's. The rate of suicide has not decreased since they became available. Antidepressants are not at fault for failing to cure all people with depression, nor are they to blame for the increased rate of suicide among young people. We live in an Age of Depression.

No one is to blame. We all did the best we can. The challenge is to do what is possible -- effectively treat those cases that can be helped.

One last analogy describes my understanding of what Ben faced in his struggle with three conditions. Helen Keller was born with two problems: she was blind and deaf. We can imagine what it would be like to become blind by putting something over our eyes. We attempt to understand deafness by blocking our ears, although this is harder to do. Living one day with those two conditions would give someone a small glimpse of what life is like with those handicaps. Even then, our appreciation for overcoming these problems is limited, because Keller was born with these conditions and had to acquire language without benefit of hearing the spoken word - an extremely difficult task.

When a child is born with three different problems: depression (distorted thinking), anxiety disorder (pervasive fearfulness), and ADHD (deficient thinking), the problems may be as difficult to deal with as were Keller's dual disabilities. It was hard for the adults in Ben's life to understand the problems he faced. It is especially incomprehensible for us when a child like Ben is intelligent, lives in a comfortable home, and attends a school with competent teachers. Keller's problems were difficult, but at least they were obvious. Children with depression, anxiety, and

ADHD are a problem for themselves and for their parents, teachers, and peers. The cause of their problems is not obvious.

As a child, Keller did finally get the specialized help that allowed her to overcome her disabilities. Finger spelling and Braille are useful tools. But if she had not been extraordinarily bright, she may not have been able to develop the potential she had. Work with young people with emotional problems must also focus on building competencies. As we build these competencies we will succeed in saving many young people who might not otherwise have been saved. In the work of helping young people with depression, anxiety, and ADHD, we may be guided by the Serenity Prayer: God grant me the serenity to accept the things I cannot change, the courage to change the things I can, and the wisdom to know the difference.

Programs like cognitive therapy, social skills training, and those methods used to cope with anxiety have great potential to help young people today. What is needed is the determination to make successful programs available to any student who chooses to have them. For students like Ben, whose conditions are severe and complex, the program may not completely solve the problem. It will, however, reduce some of the pain they suffer.

Ben's words, "You do not know what it means to me to have someone who understands," should never be forgotten.

Contents - Appendix 1

I. Screening instrument for Fourth - Sixth Grade.

II Recommended curriculum for 7th - 12th Grade

A. For Parents, Teachers, and Health Professionals

1. Psychiatric disorders of almost all suicide completers
2. Differences between suicide attempters and completers
3. Stressors preceding most adolescent suicide attempts
4. Symptom changes
5. Conditions commonly accompanying depression
6. How adolescents can help one another
7. Self-help for depressed youth

B. Especially for Health Professionals

1. Recommendations to the media -   Things to Avoid
2. Seasonal variations on suicide rates
3. General treatment goals for depressed youth
4. Crisis intervention for depressed persons
5. Modified hypoglycemic diet for persons on lithium

Note: Some of this material was obtained from a workshop presented by Dr. H. Hoberman on adolescent suicide.

I Instrument for Fourth - Sixth Grade

	Most of the time	Sometimes	Never
I look forward to things as much as I used to			
I sleep very well			
I feel like crying			
I like to go out to play			
I feel like running away			
I get stomach aches			
I have lots of energy			
I enjoy my food			
I can stick up for myself			
I think life isn't worth living			
I am good at things I do			
I enjoy the things I do as much as I used to			
I like talking with my family			
I have horrible dreams			
I feel very lonely			
I am easily cheered up			
I feel so sad I can hardly stand it			
I feel very bored			

Request for reprints to Dr. P. Birleson, The Young People's Unit, Tiperline House, Tipperline Road, Edinburgh EH105HF, U.K.

The term "depressive disorder" refers to depression that is serious enough to impairs a person's ability to function for a period of time, usually at least a number of weeks. This would exclude temporary grief reactions, normal moods shifts, demoralization, and the presence of ongoing personality traits.

Demoralization is different from pure depression disorder in that it is not as pervasive. Children who are demoralized can still enjoy themselves some of the time, sleep normally, and do not experience unusual appetite. Although they too may develop a sense of hopelessness and show signs of sadness, demoralization is often seen as either secondary to other psychiatric conditions or as a normal reaction to failure.

One can easily imagine a continuum from normal mood through demoralization to severe clinical depression. Think of another continuum with normal mood, proceeding to the common mild state of depressive that does not significantly impair functioning in one's environment, toward moderate depression which does reduce efficient functioning, ending with severe depression in which impairment is serious.

The depression scale for children was tested by comparing data from various groups of children.

1. Youngsters who were referred to the department of child psychiatry in a hospital because of clinical depression

2. Two sets of youngsters who had psychological/behavioral problems but were not diagnosed as suffering primarily from depression

3. Youngsters from a local elementary school

This self-rating instrument, by definition, does not need to be given by a psychiatrist. Because it is in the public domain, its use if not restricted. It can easily be given to any child or group of children. Because many youngsters experience depression starting as young as 4th grade, the best strategy would be to start screening then, do it several times each year, and keep a simple record of the results for future comparisons. Responses were numericalized by scoring Most of the time - 0, Sometimes - 1, Never - 2

To my knowledge there are no guidelines that differentiate the various levels of depression by specific ranges in the scores. What is known is that none of the youngsters from the local elementary school scored over 11. An examination of the data from the groups indicate that a score of 13 or above is likely to be reasonably indicative of "depressive disorder," although there may be an acceptable false positive or false negative of less than 20%.

It may be prudent to suggest that youngsters with very low scores do not experience any level of depression, and children whose scores approach 10 may suffer from mild or moderate depression. Since the ability to concentrate and remember is affected by depression, these milder forms of depression interfere with their ability to perform in school as well as their teachers, their parents, and they themselves would like. Even milder forms of depression deserve attention. Any child whose score is 11 or above should be referred to mental health professionals for further assessment.

II. Recommended Curriculum for 7th - 12th Grade

Dr. David Burns' *Ten Days To Self-Esteem* contains an easy to use depression checklist and an anxiety inventory. The scoring is easily accomplished, enabling students to see for themselves how they are doing. Burns provides a scoring key for the various levels of depression and anxiety. In the 1993 edition, a score of 0 - 4 = no depression, 5 - 10 = normal but unhappy, 11 - 20 = mild depression, 21 - 30 = moderate, 31 - 45 = severe.

Burns' text was designed as a workbook to help people who suffer from depression and anxiety. Pioneered and tested at the Presbyterian Medical Center at Philadelphia, careful research establishes its effectiveness. A leaders manual is also available, enabling classroom teachers who are willing to master this curriculum to use cognitive techniques efficiently with groups.

In the next few years I intend to publish a book entitled *Suicide Prevention: Can It Be Done?*-- a natural extension of the workshop I now present using the same title. It examines all of the factors top researchers in the field have identified as putting someone at high risk for suicide.

The content of that unpublished work is more inclusive than the chapters here that focus primarily on depression and anxiety. The new book has specific chapters on learning disabilities (especially ADHD), alcohol and drug abuse, and personality disorders (especially borderline personality and antisocial personality). It is my belief that ultimately these factors need to included in an elective class for grade 7 - 12. However, since depression and anxiety remain the single most important risk factors, the workbook *Ten Days To Self-Esteem* and the material covered here in *Depression in the Young* give a genuinely useful working foundation that will help the majority of youngsters.

A.1 PSYCHIATRIC DISORDER

Almost all suicide completers have a psychiatric disorder.

1. Depressive disorder

2. Bipolar disorder

3. Alcohol or drug abuse

4. Antisocial behavior

5. Attention Deficit-Hyperactivity Disorder

A.2 DIFFERENCES BETWEEN ADOLESCENT SUICIDE ATTEMPTERS AND COMPLETERS

1. Gender

> More females attempt than do males
> (ratio of at least 10 to 1)

> More males complete than do females
> (ratio of approximately 5 to 1)

2. Availability of firearms

Suicide completion is at least four times more likely in a home in which firearms are accessible.

A.3 STRESSORS

Attempters have two times as many negative life events in the last six months: a greater number of negative life events in their lifetime.

1. Breakup with boy/girlfriend

2. Trouble with sibling

3. Change in family financial status

4. Parents' divorce

5. Losing close friend

6. Trouble with teacher

7. Change to a new school

8. Personal illness or injury

9. Failing grades

10. Increased arguments with parents

Stressors: Loss and conflict

A.4   SYMPTOMS CHANGE AS DEPRESSED CHILDREN REACH ADOLESCENCE AND YOUNG ADULTHOOD

A. Symptoms that decrease with age

1. Depressed appearance

2. Self-esteem problems

3. Somatic complaints

4. Hallucinations

B. Symptoms that remain stable with age

1. Depressed mood

2. Poor concentration

3. Insomnia

4. Suicidal thoughts and attempts

C. Symptoms that increase with age

1. Anhedonia - (inability to experience pleasure)

2. Diurnal mood - (feeling worse in morning than later in the day)

3. Hopelessness

4. Psychomotor retardation - slowed speech

5. Definitive delusions - illogical assumptions about oneself or others

**A.5   LIST OF CONDITIONS COMMONLY
        ACCOMPANYING DEPRESSION**

Only 25% of children and adolescents have depression alone.
75% have at least one other (co-morbid) condition

A. External Disorder - problems easily seen by and
    bothersome to other people.

1. ADHD (inattention, impulsive, overactive)

2. Conduct Disorder (cannot follow rules at home or at
    school)

3. Learning Disabilities (Dyslexia - cannot read, spell or
    learn a foreign language; dyscalcula - cannot do
    math)

4. Delinquency - involvement with law enforcement

B. Internal Disorders - Problems that are internally painful to
    the person, but not necessarily troublesome to others

1. Anxiety Disorder - shortness of breath, dizziness, a
    sinking feeling in the stomach, and rapid heartbeat

2. Eating Disorder - anorexia, bulimia, obesity

3. Substance Abuse - the beginnings of alcoholism and/or
    drug addiction

A.6 HOW ADOLESCENTS CAN HELP ONE ANOTHER

1. Care about your friends; be available and listen

2. Explore possible solutions to problems, but don't tell friends what to do.

3. Try to understand without judging, arguing, denying, or minimizing feelings.

4. Tolerate depressed, irritable moods

5. Help to remember good things about them and their life.

6. Emphasize that they can live through deep hurt and that there are people who care.

7. Explore what things they can look forward to.

8. Reach out to fringe kids.

9. Maintain confidence, but if really worried about suicide, don't take chance - alert responsible adult.

A.7   SELF-HELP FOR DEPRESSED YOUTH

1. Try to understand if particular things are making you depressed.

2. Tell someone you trust how you feel - express yourself and get feelings out.

3. If necessary, write out feelings.

4. Be with other people, even if hard; avoid being alone.

5. Exercise - be physically active.

6. Do at least one thing your really enjoy, even if you don't want to do it.

7. Find something you did well or were satisfied with and praise yourself

8. Look your best.

9. Get out of the house and do something.

A.9 POSSIBLE SIGNS OF DISTRESSED YOUTH OUT OF CLASSROOM

1. Overhearing remarks indicative of significant unhappiness or despair.

2. Knowledge that prized possessions are being given away.

3. Loss of interest in extracurricular activities.

4. Direct suicide threats or attempts.

5. Marked emotionality.

6. Recent depression to suicidal behavior in family.

7. Recent conflict or losses in close relationships.

8. Increased and heavy use of alcohol or drugs

B. 1 RECOMMENDATIONS TO THE MEDIA

1. *Avoid* oversimplifying the many factors that cause the suicide

2. *Avoid* sensationalizing the suicide

3. *Avoid* glorifying the victim

4. *Avoid* making the suicide appear to be a rewarding experience or an appropriate or effective tool to achieve a personal gain

5. *Avoid* depicting the method of the suicide

6. *Avoid* emphasis to stressor or simplistic psychological presses as much as pressures

7 *Avoid* massive or repeated doses of press coverage

B 2 SEASONAL VARIATIONS ON SUICIDE RATES
Effect of light on persons with depressive illness

People who have bipolar I or major depression (typical pattern) along with impulsive/aggressive behavior are affected by rate of change in the ratio of light VS darkness. The times when change is fastest is during the spring and fall.

People who have bipolar II and others with the atypical pattern are effected by the amount of light. Summer daylight is twice as long as winter daylight. Atypical clients often have winter depression and summer hypomania. They are especially at risk during switch from depression into hypomania.

Spring has higher rate of suicide. October also shows elevated risk but not as high as March - June.

Monthly Peak Occurrences of Suicide
a review based on 61 studies (Number indicate data points)

Jan 1
Feb 1
Mar 7
April 11
May 20
June 8
July 1
Aug 1
Sep   0.5
Oct 6
Nov 3
Dec 4

B.3 GENERAL TREATMENT GOALS FOR DEPRESSED YOUTH

1. Manage immediate stressors.

2. Manage depressive symptoms.

3. Manage symptoms of co-morbid disorders.

4. Reduce impairing depressive symptoms.

5. Reduce chronic stressors, including family dysfunction and disorder.

6. Teach or enhance competencies and coping skills.

7. Deepen social relationships and expand social network.

8. Explore psychological conflicts and core pathogenic beliefs.

9. Facilitate disconfirming experiences for hopelessness and core pathogenic beliefs.

10. Create mechanisms for generalization and relapse prevention

B 4   CRISIS INTERVENTION FOR DISTRESSED PERSONS

1. Make psychological contact; establish relationship

   - create opportunity to talk privately
   - encourage talking
   - listen
   - be emphatic; communicate concern
   - clarify and summarize facts and feelings

2. Explore dimensions of crisis/problem

   - deal with immediate present
   - focus on precipitating event
   - facilitate awareness of person's reactions to stressor
   - evaluate coping (e.g., lack of inappropriate coping)
   - identify immediate needs, then eventual needs
   - access suicide risk

3. Re-conceptualize meaning of crisis

   - restate/reframe situation
   - develop linkage between low self-esteem, current stressor
   - ineffective coping, and hopelessness
   - relate crisis to problem in current roles and relationships

4. Examine possible solutions

   - what solutions already attempted
   - brainstorm other alternatives to meeting needs
   - emphasize and mobilize person's strengths and
   - competencies

5. Assist in taking specific, concrete action

   - problem-oriented and/or protection plan
   - harness existing or previously effective coping strategies
   - give advice
   - involve significant others and utilize support network

6. Follow-up
   - contract
   - arrange procedure
   - emphasize caring

B 5   MODIFIED HYPOGLYCEMIC DIET FOR PERSONS ON LITHIUM

The recommendations here are generally applicable for persons who experience weight gain on lithium. Specific recommendations for individuals should be obtained by a dietitian in cooperation with physician orders.

1. Avoid simple (refined) carbohydrates that involve high levels of sugar,

2. Increase complex carbohydrates such as breads, cereals and vegetables,

3. Increase high fiber foods such as fruits, vegetables and grains,

4. Decrease fat in your diet,

5. Eat a number of small meals and healthy snacks between meals.

NOTE:

This short list sounds like everything you have been hearing in the last years about what constitutes a healthy diet to decrease the risk of heart disease and cancer. Consequently, the person on lithium simply needs to eat a generally healthy diet.

WORKS CITED

Adolescent stress and depression. (1986). Teens in distress. University of Minnesota: Minnesota Extension Service.

Ardrey, R. (1961). African genesis: A personal investigation into the animal origins and nature of man. New York: Dell Publishing Co., Inc.

Burns, D.D., M.D. (1980). Feeling good: The new mood therapy. New York: Signet Books.

Campbell, J. (1990). Transformations of myth through time. New York: Harper & Row.

Campbell Joseph & Bill Moyer, (1988), The Power of Myth. New York: Doubleday Dell Publishing Group Inc.

Diagnostic and Statistical Manual of Mental Disorders, Fourth Edition (1994) Washington DC: American Psychiatric Association.

Fawcett, J.A., MD (1991). Understanding the new risk factors for suicide. Lifesavers: The Newsletter of the American Suicide Foundation, 3:3.

Fawcett, J.A., MD (1992). Short- and long-term predictors of suicide in depressed patients. Lifesavers: The Newsletter of the American Suicide Foundation.

Fieve, F.R., MD (1975). Moodswings. New York: Bantam Books.

Fishman, K.D. (1991, June). Therapy for children. The Atlantic Monthly, pp. 47-69.

Gawain, S. (1978). Creative Visualizations. New York: Bantam Books.

Gelman, D. (1987, May 4). Depression. Newsweek. pp. 48-57.

Gold, M.S. (1987). The good news about depression. New York:
    Bantam Books.

Goode, E. (1990, March 5). Beating depression. U.S. News & World
    Report, pp. 48-55.

Hoberman, H.M., Ph.D. (1989). Completed suicide in children and
    adolescents: A review. In B.D. Garfinkel (Ed.), Adolescent
    suicide: Recognition, treatment, and prevention. New York:
    Haworth.

Jamison, K. (1994) Suicide and Manic-Depressive Illness, Lifesavers:
    The Newsletter of the American Suicide Foundation. 6:3

Klerman, G., Weissman, M., Rounsaville, B., & Chevron, E. (1984).
    Interpersonal psychotherapy of depression. New York: Basic
    Books, Inc.

McKay, M. & Fanning, P. (1987). Self esteem. Oakland, California:
    New Harbinger Publications.

McKnew, D.H., Cytryn, L., & Yahraes, H. (1983). Why isn't Johnny
    crying? Coping with depression in children. New York:
    Norton & Company.

Physicians' Desk Reference (1993) Montvale, N.J.: Medical Economics
    Company Inc.

Popper, C., MD (1989). Diagnosing bipolar vs. ADHD, American
    Academy of Child and Adolescent Psychiatry News.
    Washington DC

Roy, A., (1992). Schizophrenia and suicide. Lifesavers: The Newsletter
    of the American Suicide Foundation.

Sargent, M. (1989 a). Depressive illnesses: Treatment brings new
    hope. U.S. Department of Health and Human Services.
    National Institute of Mental Health.

152

Sheehan, D.V. (1983). The anxiety disease. New York: Bantam Books.

Stevens, A. (1989). The roots of war: A Jungian perspective. New York: Paragon House.

Supporting young people following a suicide. (1986) Teens in distress. University of Minnesota: Minnesota Extension Service.

Understanding the new risk factors for suicide. (1991, Summer). Lifesavers: The Newsletter of the American Suicide Foundation.

Useful information on suicide. (1986). U.S. Department of Health and Human Services. National Institute of Mental Health.

Weissman, M., Ph.D. (1991). Panic and suicidal behavior. Lifesavers: The Newsletter of the American Suicide Foundation.

IMPORTANT ADDRESSES

American Foundation For Suicide Prevention
120 Wall Street, 22nd Floor
New York, NY 10005
(212)410-1111

The Compassionate Friends
P.O. Box 3696
Oak Brook, IL 60522-3696

American Association of Suicidology
Suite 310
4201 Connecticut Ave., NW
Washington, DC 20008

Friends for Survival Inc.
P. O. Box 214463
Sacramento, CA 95821

FURTHER REFERENCES

Beck, Rush, Shaw and Emery, Cognitive Therapy of Depression (1979) Guilford Press, New York.

Elmer-Dewitt, P. (1992, July 6). Depression: The growing role of drug therapies. Time, pp. 57-59.

Gorman, J.M., MD (1990) The Essential Guide to Psychiatric Drugs. New York: St. Martin's Press.

Hewett, J.H. (1980). After suicide. Philadelphia, Pennsylvania: The Westminster Press.

Kubler-Ross, Elisabeth. (1975). Death, the final growth stage. Prentice-Hall, Inc., Englewood Cliff, NJ

Larson, D.E., MD (Ed.). (1990). Mayo Clinic family health book. New York: William Morrow and Company, Inc.

Sargent, M. (1990). Helping the depressed person get treatment. U.S. Department of Health and Human Services. National Institute of Mental Health.

Sarnoff Schiff, H. (1977). The bereaved parent. NY: Penguin Books.

Supporting distressed young people. (1985). Teens in distress. University of Minnesota: Minnesota Extension Service.

Teen suicide. (1985). Teens in distress. University of Minnesota: Minnesota Extension Service.

Veninga, R.L. (1985). A gift of hope: How we survive our tragedies. New York: Ballantine Books.

Wrobleski, A. (1991). Suicide survivors: A guide for those left behind. Minneapolis, Minnesota: Afterwords Publishing.

Youth Suicide Prevention Programs: A Resource Guide, National Center for Injury Prevention and Control, Centers for Disease Control, Mailstop F-36, 4770 Buford Highway NE, Atlanta, GA 30341

INDEX

ABOUT THE AUTHOR

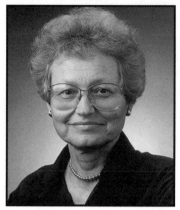 Trudy Carlson never intended to write this book. Yet the death of her son Ben forced her put aside other works in order to the story of his life and death. She began to record everything she'd observed during the his life, including the steps the family took to help him obtain treatment and understand his condition.

As she wrote she discovered three distinct topics. The first became the book, The Suicide of My Son: A Story of Childhood Depression. This is now also published as two separate works: Ben's Story and Depression in the Young.

Learning Disabilities: How to Recognize & Manage Learning & Behavioral Problems in Children contrasts Ben's ADD (Attention Deficit Disorder) with her own personal struggle with a mild case of dyslexia. She explains why she was able to manage her problems, and why Ben's were overwhelming.

Tragedy, Finding a Hidden Meaning: How to Transform the Tragedies in Your Life into Personal Growth, explores the personal and spiritual growth that can emerge from loss. "Meaning makes most things endurable, perhaps everything."

Suicide Survivors Handbook: A Guide for the Bereaved and Those Who Wish to Help Them, deals with the major issues confronting the survivor. It also gives a wealth of practical suggestions on what is most helpful during recovery from grief.

ORDER FORM

Telephone orders: Call Toll Free: 1-800-296-7163
Have your Visa or MasterCard number ready
Postal Orders: Benline Press, 118 N. 60th Ave. E.
Duluth, MN 55804
Please send the following books. I understand that I may return any books for a full refund -- for any reason, no questions asked.

Suicide Survivor's Handbook: A Guide to the Bereaved and
Those Who Wish to Help Them $14.95 _____

Ben's Story: The Symptoms of Depression, ADHD and
Anxiety that Caused His Suicide $9.95 _____

Tragedy, Finding a Hidden Meaning: How to Transform
the Tragedies in Your Life into Personal Growth $14.95 _____

Learning Disabilities: How to Recognize and Manage
Learning and Behavioral Problems in Children $14.95 _____

Sales Tax: Please add 6.5% for books shipped to Minnesota addresses.

_____

Shipping: Book Rate: $2.00 for the first book and 75 cents for
each additional book. (Surface shipping may take three
to four weeks)   Airmail: $3.50 per book.

Total   _____

Payment: __ check __ credit card
Card Number:_____
Name on card:_____Exp. Date _____/_____